The Ultima
to Eat-St

MW00930508

Table of Contents

Introduction

The Eat-Stop-Eat protocol is one of several intermittent fasting methods that have helped many people lose excess body weight and, in the process, improve their general health. It's also one of the most popular protocols because it's one of the simplest and most flexible of the current intermittent fasting protocols. And in this book, you will get the opportunity to learn what the protocol really is about, the science behind weight loss, and how to optimally implement this protocol. By the end of the book, you will be in a very good position to start the Eat-Stop-Eat protocol armed with all the knowledge you'll need to do so.

So, if you're ready, turn the page and let's begin!

Chapter 1 – Fasting and Weight Loss

Chances are, the primary reason you want to fast intermittently using the Eat-Stop-Eat protocol (ESE for brevity) is to lose weight. While doing the protocol right is enough to help you lose weight, that won't be as fun as understanding how intermittent fasting protocols, like the ESE, can help you lose weight. So before diving right into the protocol, let's talk about how fasting helps people lose weight.

Weight Loss 101

To clearly understand how people lose and gain weight, one must have an idea of how the human body utilizes energy.

The human body is either in a fasted or a fed state. While in a fed state, the pancreas produces and releases more of the hormone called insulin into the bloodstream. Different types of foods trigger different levels of insulin production except for one kind of food: dietary fat.

Insulin can be thought of as a nutrient antenna or sensor. It's because insulin is able to "sense" when the human body ingests carbohydrates or protein-rich foods. Simple carbohydrates, which are abundant in refined foods, are the types of food that trigger the highest level of insulin production in the body.

For the human body to perform basic functions that are crucial for survival, like breathing, heart beating, detoxification via the kidneys and liver, or thinking, it needs a continuous energy source. But because it isn't possible to continuously ingest calories from food for energy, the body uses an energy storage system to provide itself the energy it needs when food isn't available. Energy can be stored in 2 ways: in the liver as glycogen and all over the body as body fat.

Many people wrongly assume that weight loss is but a simple and compartmentalized issue. In other words, they make the mistake of thinking excess calories or energy can be stored in just one area of the body and later on, withdrawn from the same area. It's like leaving your car keys in your drawer and when you need it later, you retrieve it from that drawer.

The entire weight loss-weight gain mechanism can be summarized by a simple mathematical equation that even kindergarten students can understand. That equation is:

Body Fat = Calories Consumed − Calories Burned

This is the main foundation of weight loss. All diets and programs aimed at helping people lose excess weight, especially body fat, are founded on this principle. And this principle is inviolable.

Looking at the equation, weight gain, whether in the form of muscles or body fat, happens when a person consistently consumes more calories than what his or her body can burn throughout the day. On the other hand, weight loss happens when a person consistently burns more calories than what he or she consumes daily.

You can think of gaining or losing weight in the same manner as you think about your bank account. If you spend more than you earn, you continue losing money or worse, going into debt. In the same manner, spending more calories than you earn daily is the key to successful weight loss.

Let's go back to the misconception of energy being stored only in one area of the body and being "withdrawn" only through the same area. Given the equation above, a person can maintain his or her bodyweight if they consume an average of 2,000 calories daily while burning roughly the same amount. And if that person wants to lose weight, he or she will need to reduce calories believing that the caloric deficit will be made up for by his or her stored body fat in order to successfully lose weight.

Right? Well, not exactly. Why?

Again, the belief that energy can only be stored in one area or "container" of the body and can be withdrawn only through that area or container is an inaccurate one. This is because the body stores excess energy in two places: the liver (as glycogen) and key areas of the body (as body fat) like the tummy, butt, thighs, arms, or face. While stored energy can be stored in these 2 areas, a person can withdraw energy from one source at a time only. Allow me to illustrate.

Think of driving on a wide road and you're approaching a fork on that road. When you get to the fork, the only way to continue moving forward is to choose between the two dissecting roads in front of you: the left or the right. When you choose the left, you can't drive on the right and vice versa.

You can imagine the human body getting its energy in the same way. If it gets energy from the food that it's eating at the moment, it won't be able to tap into its stored energy reserves, i.e., body fat or glycogen. When a person eats food, his or her pancreas produces insulin. And when he or she eats simple carbohydrates, the higher the amount of insulin the pancreas produces.

And this is where the concern lies: insulin can prevent the body from using stored energy, i.e., body fat or glycogen. In case you're interested, the metabolic processes used to refer to using body fat and glycogen for energy are lipolysis and glycogenesis, respectively.

For the average person, eating 3 meals a day is standard operating procedure. But eating meals is only possible during one's waking hours. What happens during sleep at night? It's called fasting.

Fasting – or a fasted state – is when a person doesn't eat. And because nobody eats in their sleep, which can't be said for talking or walking, everybody fasts during the night when asleep.

During a fasted state, the pancreas doesn't produce insulin and as such, insulin levels drop. But because the important metabolic processes necessary to stay alive continue (heart beating, breathing, etc.) even while asleep, the body continues to need energy. Since there's no food to get energy, the body will get its energy requirements from stored energy either in the form of glycogen or body fat. And because insulin is very low, there's nothing to inhibit lipolysis and glycogenesis in the body.

When a person fasts, i.e., deliberately goes without food for extended periods of time, he or she enters into a fasted state where insulin levels fall. By fasting, a person can turn to his or her body's stored energy. The first energy source tapped by the body during fasted states is the liver, i.e., glycogen. When glycogen levels are depleted, the body then turns to body fat for its energy requirements.

To summarize the human body's energy sources, it's food, then glycogen, and finally body fat. To lose weight, therefore, a person needs to exhaust energy from food and glycogen before he or she's able to burn body fat.

When a person fasts for an extended period of time, say 24 hours, his or her body will demand the average daily caloric requirement that wasn't available from food. Because an obese or overweight person has abundant supply of stored body fat, his or her body can "claim" the average daily caloric balance or deficit from body fat. It's as if that person's body will say, "Take in as much fat as you want! I'm swimming in it anyway!"

Either the human body stores fat or burns it up. It's one or the other – it's impossible to do both simultaneously. The human body's more intelligent than most people think. When food is abundant, it stores energy and when food is scarce, it will run to stored energy such as glycogen and body fat for energy.

Insulin calls the shots in terms of where the body will get its energy from food or stored energy. If you want to turn on your body's fat burning mode, turn the insulin-producing switch off.

Many people still adhere to the 6-small-meals-daily method for losing weight. While it's an effective way to lose body fat, it's not the optimal way of doing it. Why? Because by eating frequently, especially carbohydrates like pasta, rice, and bread, the pancreas is compelled to produce insulin and depending on the kinds of calories consumed, insulin levels can spike and prevent glycogenesis and lipolysis.

While caloric reduction is the underlying principle for weight loss, it's not as simple as simply eating less calories than what you consume. How you achieve caloric deficits is equally important. By reducing calories through intermittent fasting, you minimize your body's production of insulin and optimize its glycogenesis and lipolysis processes. When you consistently achieve lipolysis, you can consistently burn body fat and eventually, lose excess weight.

And that, my friend, is how intermittent fasting can help you lose excess body fat and consequently, excess weight.

Things to Know about the 5:2 Diet

5:2 is a popular method used by people who want to lose weight. The principle of this diet is quite simple- eat like you normally do for five days in a week, and for the other two days, you are required to consume between 500 to 600 calories. Here are a couple of things that you must understand about this diet.

Please don't consider the meaning of the word "fasting" in its literal sense. Don't be under any misconception that you are free to eat for five days and then must abstain from food on the other two days. Instead of abstaining from food, you merely need to cut down on your calorie intake. You must fast for two days, but never schedule the fasting period on two consecutive days. Your body needs the energy to sustain itself and function optimally. If you drastically reduce your food intake for over 48-hours, then you run the risk of burning yourself out. If you don't want to experience fatigue, then plan the week such that the fasting days aren't consecutive.

Yes, you can eat like you normally do for five days in a given week, but you must not think of these days as cheat days. You will not be able to see a positive change in your overall health if you keep binging on unhealthy foods for five days in a week and then fast for two days. The calorie restriction on the two days of fast will not be effective if you aren't mindful of your diet on the other days. When you consume healthy and wholesome meals, it will not only help with weight loss, but it will also prevent fatigue. If you overeat or compensate for the fasting days on the other days, then the diet cannot be effective.

A basic idea that applies to all aspects of life is "everything in moderation." This rule applies to diet as well. If weight loss is your goal, then you need to maintain a calorie deficit. To attain and maintain a calorie deficit, you must reduce your calorie intake, increase your calorie expenditure (exercise or through any other physical activity) or follow a combination of both. With the 5:2 diet protocols, you can effectively reduce your overall calorie intake by fasting for two days. Don't push your body too much and remember the "everything in moderation" rule. Too much or too little of anything is undesirable and keep this in mind while planning your week for the 5:2 diet.

You need to ensure that you don't deprive your body of the necessary nutrients it needs. A nutritional deficiency can harm your health and hinder the process of weight loss. So, you must never eliminate entire food groups from your diet. That said, you could certainly reduce your intake of certain foods like carbs and sugars to improve your overall health.

A healthy adult can safely follow the protocols of intermittent fasting. However, some must not diet like pregnant or lactating women, individuals who underwent surgery recently or might undergo one shortly, those who dealt with or have any eating disorders, and those who are ill.

Keep in mind that it will take your body a while to get used to this pattern of eating. You might experience mood swings or fluctuations in your energy levels. These things are quite common and will slowly disappear as your body starts getting used to the 5:2diet. In the meanwhile, it is quintessential that you stick to the diet and don't give up. A little patience and resilience are important.

You will need to change your mindset about dieting. When you are dieting, don't think that you are depriving yourself of some foods. Instead, you must think that you are providing your body with the nutrition it needs. A change in diet is as much a physical change as a psychological one. If you feel that you are depriving yourself of food, the chances of binging on foods will increase. Also, it will become rather difficult to stick to the diet. Before you make any dietary changes, you must always consult your health care provider about the same.

Intermittent Fasting and Autophagy

Intermittent fasting helps with calorie restriction and also induces mild ketosis. It means that it is quite easy to limit your calorie intake, and it prompts your body to start burning fats to provide energy. There is another major health benefit that intermittent fasting offers, and it is autophagy. However, before learning about autophagy and how helpful it is, it is important to learn about apoptosis.

The death of an organism is not a single event but a combination of smaller events that eventually leads to its death. This death is quintessential for life, for a new life at least. Wait, does this sound too ominous?

All living organisms consist of a large and complicated network of cellular structures. The cells within the organisms tend to get damaged from time and time and die. This takes place within our bodies too. It is important that the old and damaged cells are wiped out to accommodate new and healthy cells. This is an ongoing process and is quintessential to maintain your optimal health. Are you wondering why these cells die? Cells, at times, get damaged because of various external factors such as injuries, infections, or even due to the buildup of toxins. For instance, whenever you cut your finger, the blood supply to some cells gets cut off, and these cells eventually die. This process is referred to as necrosis.

At times, cells get damaged even due to the regular wear and tear. When this happens, your body takes steps to kill those cells to help the growth of healthier cells through a process known as apoptosis. As ominous as it all sounds, apoptosis is essential for a healthy body. For instance, did you know that a fetus has webbed feet while in the womb? The webbing disappears over time, and fingers appear. The cells used in the webbing are removed through apoptosis. The brain tends to create several millions of neurons initially, but only some of them become a part of the neural pathways responsible for the creation of our thoughts and memories. The rest of the unused neurons die voluntarily through apoptosis.

The best way to understand apoptosis is to think of the human body as a company that rents out equipment. There are several millions of cells that are present within the form of equipment it rents out. To go ahead with this analogy, you are merely a tenant in your body and have a contract with the rental company. Whenever you need to perform a specific task, the company will provide you with access codes to certain machinery that you need to accomplish the task. For instance, if you want to lift a bottle, your body will mobilize the cells in your fingers to help you lift the bottle. Even when you want to run, your body mobilizes all the muscle fibers to help you complete the run.

After a while, like all equipment, even this one is susceptible to the damage of regular wear and tear. If the equipment is damaged, it cannot perform like it is supposed to. Remember that your body takes this agreement rather seriously. If you keep up your end of the bargain and provide your body with the fuel that it needs, then it will make sure that you get good service. However, optimum performance cannot be guaranteed if the cells within are damaged. So, your body continuously performs internal quality checks and determines the cells that need to be repaired and those that must be removed. As mentioned, the removal of damaged cells is referred to as apoptosis. The cells that can be repaired are fixed through a process known as autophagy.

Autophagy is derived from a Greek word, which roughly translates to mean, "Eat oneself." Let us continue with the previous analogy, assume that your body just performed a quality check, and it was noticed that a cell had been damaged. Almost like a car that needs a wheel alignment or an oil refill. Instead of servicing the entire car, it makes sense to work on the issue that must be fixed. Likewise, even your body starts to repair that specific cell which was damaged. During this repair, if there are any parts that cannot be salvaged, then they will be removed, and any important portions of such part will be used in the manufacture of a new part.

Autophagy is similar to car servicing, and this cannot take place if the car is still being used, can it? If you need to get the car serviced, you will need to take it to the garage and leave it there so the mechanic can start working on it. The same applies to your body if you want autophagy to work.

For instance, if you keep consuming food, then your insulin levels stay high, and your body cannot initiate this process of "self-service." So, for autophagy to kick in, there needs to be a reduction in your calorie intake.

Chapter 2 – The Eat-Stop-Eat Intermittent Fasting Protocol

Now that you have an idea of the mechanism by which intermittent fasting can help you lose weight, it's time to sink your teeth into the Eat-Stop-Eat protocol.

Developed by nutrition and weight-loss expert Brad Pilon, the main idea underlying the ESE protocol is when you eat is much more important than what you eat when you're trying to lose excess weight. According to Pilon, there are numerous scientific researches that support the idea that intermittent fasting, or regularly avoiding food for extended periods of time, is much better in terms of losing body fat and retaining muscle mass compared to diets that simply reduce caloric intake or avoid specific types of food.

How It Works

Implementing this protocol is fairly simple: eat normally for 5 to 6 days during the week and fast for 1 or 2 days only. Each fasting session should at least be 20 hours straight and it's best if you do it for 24 hours. So if your last meal was at 7 am today, your next meal should be between 3 am (20 hours) and 7 am (24 hours) the following morning. Also, you shouldn't schedule your fasting sessions on consecutive days. For optimal results, put at least a day in between your weekly fasting sessions.

During your fasting days, you shouldn't consume any calories, which means you'll need to stick to calorie-free beverages only. These include plain water, unsweetened natural teas, and unsweetened black coffee. If you want some taste, you can use calorie-free sugar substitutes like aspartame or stevia on your tea or coffee.

By fasting at least once weekly, Brad Pilon claims that it's possible for you to create a 10% caloric deficit for the week. If you go for twice weekly, you can achieve a 20% caloric deficit and greater body fat and weight loss.

On your normal eating days, take note of the word "normal." This means you should eat the same amount of food that allowed you to maintain your body weight just prior to implementing the ESE protocol. Normal eating doesn't mean binge or over-eating because it will just make your body recoup the caloric deficit and fat loss it accomplishes during the fasting days. When that happens, you don't lose body fat and can even gain more!

During your eating days, nothing's off the table...literally. You can eat pretty much anything you were eating prior to going on the ESE protocol in the amounts that allowed you to maintain your weight. Again, eating normally is different from overeating, ok?

How's It Different from the 5:2 Diet?

On the surface, the 5:2 diet and Eat-Stop-Eat look the same. However, they're not. Here are the key differences distinguishing the two:

- Definition of Fasting: With the 5:2 diet, fasting isn't defined as completely avoiding calories but limiting caloric consumption for the day to 800 calories maximum. With the Eat-Stop-Eat protocol, fasting means complete abstinence from calories for 24 hours. Thus, the 5:2 diet is the relatively easier diet between the two.

- Calorie-Counting: The 5:2 diet requires that you count the calories of the foods you eat, particularly on fasting days. Hence, you'll need to carefully measure what you eat on those days to ensure that you don't exceed the 800-calorie daily limit. But with Eat-Stop-Eat, you're not required to count calories. Why? It's because there's nothing to count since you shouldn't even be getting any calories for the day! This makes the 5:2 diet mentally more complicated than Eat-Stop-Eat.
- Fasting Frequency: The 5:2 diet requires 2 non-consecutive days of fasting every week. Otherwise, it'd be the 4-to-5:1-to-2 diet. Eat-Stop-Eat on the other hand, gives you an option to fast for just 1 day a week or for 2 non-consecutive days. We can't say that the 5:2 diet's harder on the basis of the 2 non-consecutive fasting day requirement because you can eat during your fasting days. It's also hard to conclude that Eat-Stop-Eat's harder because even if you have the option of fasting just once per week, you can't eat anything with calories on that single fasting day. So, I guess it's a tie in terms of difficulty!

Why the Eat-Stop-Eat Works

During fasted states, the body's external energy source – a.k.a. Food – is non-existent. Because the body doesn't get any energy externally, it's forced to go inside for it. It has no choice but to tap on its energy reserves. It goes for glycogen first and when it's depleted, it starts to use body fat for energy.

While it's a very efficient way to lose body fat, too much of a good thing can become bad too. When you fast for too long, your body will start turning to meat instead of fat for energy. What this means is your body will start to use your muscles for energy, i.e., muscle catabolism.

Why do you need to learn this? Metabolism, which is the rate at which the body burns calories or body fat, is largely determined by the amount of muscle mass a person has. The more muscle mass, the faster the metabolism and vice versa.

Over-fasting can eat away significant muscle mass. When that happens, metabolism slows down. When metabolism slows down, a person's ability to burn lose body fat declines and fat loss plateaus.

This is the reason why crash and extremely restrictive diets quickly stop working. At first, crash diets lead to substantial weight loss, but over time, it leads to serious muscle catabolism. When metabolism slows down substantially, extreme dieters think they need to further reduce their already extremely-reduced calories. By then, their metabolism has slowed down so much that further fat and weight loss is no longer possible.

One of the strengths of the Eat-Stop-Eat protocol is that you avoid over-fasting, which means you also avoid muscle catabolism. When you're able to maintain your muscle mass, you maintain your metabolism and you can continue burning body fat. Even better, you can increase your metabolism if you're able to increase muscle mass through the right exercises.

In other words, the fasting duration and frequency of the Eat-Stop-Eat is such that it's long enough to put your body in fat-burning mode and sustain it, and short enough to avoid muscle catabolism. Thus, the Eat-Stop-Eat protocol is one of the best ways to strip off body fat without suffering a significant loss in muscle mass.

Implementing the Protocol

When you start implementing the protocol, here are some of the key things you'll need to do:

- Fast 1 to 2 days every week on non-consecutive days, where you don't consume any calories for 20 to 24 hours straight;
- You can drink calorie-free beverages on your fasting days, e.g., plain water, unsweetened tea or black coffee, or stevia/calorie-free-sweetener sweetened tea or black coffee;
- You can also chew on sugar-free and zero-calorie gum during your fasting days because the whole point is to avoid calories only;
- When you start fasting, take baby steps by limiting your fasting duration to what you can realistically do and gradually increase your fasting time over the succeeding weeks or months to avoid shocking yourself out of the protocol.
- Don't break your fasts with huge meals but with regular-sized ones only; and
- On your regular eating days, eat normally, i.e., the same amount you did to maintain your weight prior to implementation of the protocol.

Food List

In this section, you will learn about the different foods you can eat while following the protocols of intermittent fasting.

Even while you are fasting, the most important thing is always to keep your body hydrated. The amount of water your body needs will differ from one person to another. However, as a general rule of thumb, you need to drink eight glasses (8 oz each) of water per day. The best way to check whether you are hydrated or not is to check the color of your urine. If it is pale yellow or clear, it means your body is hydrated and dark yellow is an indication of dehydration. Dehydration can also cause fatigue, headaches, and lightheadedness. Dehydration, coupled with a decrease in your calorie intake, can harm your body. If you want, you can always spruce up the drinking water by adding a few sprigs of mint, slices of cucumber or even lime to the water.

Avocado is a super-food that you must include in your diet. You might be wondering why it is a good idea to add a high-calorie fruit to your diet when you want to lose weight. Well, avocados contain monounsaturated fats, and these are good for your metabolism and health. Adding half an avocado to your meal can make you feel fuller for longer.

Fish contains proteins as well as healthy fats along with traces of Vitamin D. Try to include fish into your diet as often as you can. This lean protein will give your body the necessary nutrients without adding onto your calorie intake. While selecting fish, opt for naturally fatty fish like salmon, mackerel, and trout. Also, whenever possible, opt for fish caught in the wild instead of the factory-farmed varieties.

Different foods like broccoli, cauliflower, and Brussels sprouts are full of dietary fiber. By including cruciferous vegetables to your diet, you can improve your digestion and prevent constipation. Also, fibrous foods will leave you feeling fuller for longer since your body takes a while to digest them.

There is a popular misconception that when it comes to food, all white foods are bad. Well, this is just a misconception, and you must not read much into it. One food you must try to include in your diet in limited quantities is a potato. Potatoes are good for your health, but it doesn't mean you binge on French fries or chips. A baked potato with different fixings can be a filling meal.

Beans and legumes are a great way to include complex carbs to your meals, and they aren't calorie dense. For instance, foods like black beans, lentils, chickpeas, and peas can help with weight loss even while you are on a calorie restriction. So, if you love chili or hummus, then you don't have to give up on them while following the protocols of the 5:2 diet.

Did you know that your gut is home to millions of microbes? Most of these microbes are helpful and help improve your body's ability to digest and absorb food. However, you need to take care of these microbes, or they can wreak havoc on your health. The best source of nutrition for the gut microbiome is probiotic foods. Probiotics like kefir, sauerkraut, kombucha, and yogurt can be added to your diet.

You can add all sorts of berries to your diet. Berries like strawberries, cherries, blackberries, raspberries, blueberries and so on are rich in antioxidants and vitamin C. Also, berries make for a great dessert or snack, especially when you are limiting your calorie intake.

One egg has about six grams of protein in it and contains only about 80 calories. Try to include eggs to your diet, and your body's protein needs will be taken care of. Apart from this, they are quite easy to cook too.

Include different types of nuts like pistachios, walnuts, and almonds along with different seeds like sunflower, chia, and flax seeds to your diet. Nuts and seeds contain healthy polyunsaturated fats and dietary fiber, which are good for your health.

Include whole grains like farro, amaranth, sorghum, bulgur, spelt, or even freekeh to your diet. Whole grains are full of protein and fiber. Even eating one portion of whole grains in a meal can leave you feeling quite full.

Meal Plan Ideas

The main component of the 5:2 diet is that you are required to consume between 500 to 600 calories on fasting days. Therefore, it is quintessential that you consume foods that are not only nutrient-dense but are filling too. At times, you might not have a lot of time to cook on the weekdays, so having a pre-planned menu will help get through such days while maintaining the diet. To ease the stress of prepping for a diet, here are ten meal plan ideas you can use. All the different recipes given in this chapter are around the 500-calorie limit set by the diet.

Day One

Breakfast: One sachet of Quaker Oats porridge (255 calories)

Dinner: Beetroot and feta salad with baby spinach leaves (125 calories)

Snack: Sliced apples served with a tablespoon of almond butter (145 calories)

Day Two

Breakfast: Sweet plums and unsweetened natural yogurt (140 calories).

Dinner: 2 pieces of wholegrain cracker breads with tuna slices and rocket leaves (255 calories)

Snack: A bowl of miso soup (35 calories).

Day Three

Breakfast: One soft-boiled egg with five pieces of asparagus (90 calories).

Dinner: One turkey burger with a portion of corn on the cob (320 calories)

Snack: Handful of frozen grapes (60 calories).

Day Four

Breakfast: A sachet of muesli or a packet of Belvita Breakfast biscuits (225 calories)

Dinner: Roasted vegetables like courgette, aubergine, red pepper, and butternut squash served with a balsamic glaze (250 calories).

Snack: A bowl of miso soup (35 calories)

Day Five

Breakfast: 2-egg omelet with baby spinach leaves (160 calories)

Dinner: 40 grams of hummus and a medium bowl of crudités (180 calories)

Snack: Edamame beans sprinkled with rock salt (85 calories)

Day Six

Breakfast: One banana with 100 grams of low-fat, unsweetened natural yogurt (180 calories)

Dinner: A portion of grilled turkey breast with spinach leaves (215 calories)

Snack: 10 grams of salted popcorn (60 calories).

Day Seven

Breakfast: Apple, ginger and carrot smoothie without any sweeteners (105 calories)

Dinner: Whole meal pita pizza with tomatoes, herbs and a little cheese (180 calories)

Snack: A handful of almonds and 100 grams of blueberries (140 calories).

Day Eight

Breakfast: A mixed berry bowl of 100 grams each of strawberries, raspberries, and blueberries (115 calories).

Dinner: Harissa grilled chicken with vegetable couscous (315 calories)

Snack: Around ten pistachios (60 calories)

Day Nine

Breakfast: Buttermilk pancakes (200 calories)

Dinner: Roasted tomato and red pepper soup with multigrain crackers (130 calories)

Snack: One tablespoon each of pumpkin and sunflower seeds (90 calories).

Day Ten

Breakfast: 50 grams of muesli (190 calories)

Dinner: Grilled fillet of salmon served with pesto and steamed kale leaves (295 calories)

Snack: a handful of cherries (25 calories)

You can mix things up a little and come up with your own variations, but having certain meal ideas ready will come in handy.

Important Nutrients to Concentrate On

Intermittent fasting has been gaining popularity rapidly in the last couple of years, and it seems to have become a buzzword in the world of fitness and health. However, it is so much more than a buzzword. A lot of people opt to follow intermittent fasting to improve their overall health and physical wellbeing. In this section, you will learn about the different supplements you can take to ensure your body is getting all the nutrients it needs to function optimally.

Creatine

One of the most popular supplements that help with gaining muscle mass and promoting muscle growth is creatine. Creatine is a natural monohydrate present within the cells in a muscle. A lot of athletes take creatine supplements to enhance their performance. Whenever you take creatine supplements, your body tends to expand its phosphocreatine stores- a type of stored energy present within the cells, which helps your body synthesize more adenosine triphosphate (ATP). ATP helps your body get the necessary energy it needs for optimal performance during exercising. The best time to take a creatine supplement is while you are fasting since your body absorbs it better.

Collagen

Another popular supplement available these days is collagen. It is one of the most abundant sources of protein in your body. Collagen is present in your skin, in the muscles, connective tissues, tendons, and ligaments too. Your body does synthesize collagen on its own, but as you age, the production of collagen tends to slow down. It is quintessential that you include collagen supplements if you want your skin to retain its elasticity, supply the necessary structure to tendons and joints, and maintain an optimal supply of protein to the organs. If you are limiting your calorie intake, as you would while following the 5:2 diet, then it is important to include collagen supplements.

Zinc

An important nutrient your body needs is zinc. However, this nutrient isn't synthesized in your body. A zinc supplement is suitable for everyone, regardless of their dietary habits and lifestyle. Zinc helps with the synthesis of proteins; it is essential for growth and development of the body, the production of DNA, maintenance of the immune system, and for healing wounds. Zinc supplements don't usually have any added calories, and you must take them while in a fasted state. Also, if your diet is usually rich in shellfish, then you don't usually need any zinc supplements. You must not consume over 30mg of zinc per day.

Amino acids

Amino acids help stimulate the synthesis of proteins in the body for building muscle and preventing the breakdown of muscles while in a calorie deficit. Consuming branched chain amino acids or BCAAs while fasting can break the fast since you will be consuming a form of protein. However, while following the protocols of the 5:2 diet, you don't have to worry about breaking the fast since you never really abstain yourself from eating. The best time to consume BCAAs is before you start exercising since it helps increase the flow of energy in your muscles and increases the efficiency of exercising.

Caffeine

You can consume coffee if you want. However, while following the 5:2 diet, you must ensure your calorie intake on the fast days doesn't exceed 500 calories. So, you can consume coffee with all the fixings only if your calorie allowance provides for it. The best option is to consume black coffee without sugar and cream or even herbal teas. Caffeine can make you feel energized and refreshed. Beverages like tea and coffee tend to have a diuretic effect on your body, so you must ensure you don't consume too much of it. Also, avoid consuming caffeine late in the day because it can make it difficult to fall asleep if you keep experiencing caffeine jitters. Most of the pre-workout supplements tend to contain caffeine to promote the efficiency of the workout.

Sodium

Sodium is the most important electrolyte your body needs to function optimally. While you are fasting, you must supplement your body with the electrolytes it needs. Electrolytes are the chemicals, which are quintessential for basic functions like transmission of nerve impulses, firing of neurons, regulating blood pressure, and for muscle contractions. If you ever feel dehydrated while fasting, it is most likely due to the lack of sodium. There are different sodium supplements you can take. However, the best dietary source of sodium is salt. So, ensure that you include sufficient salt in all your meals.

Vitamin D

This is also referred to as the sunshine vitamin since it is manufactured in the body after it is exposed to the rays of the sun. Vitamin D essentially helps in balancing calcium in the body. A deficiency in vitamins can lead to several issues like obesity, diabetes, hypertension, cardiac arrest, stroke, and even muscle weakness. Men who don't spend much time in the sun might not be able to get the necessary vitamin D from the food they eat. The only food sources of vitamin D are egg yolks, fortified milk, naturally fatty fish, and fortified cereals.

Potassium

Potassium is another electrolyte that your body needs to function properly. It helps stabilize your blood pressure and keep up your heart's health. Potassium is a mineral that most individuals don't get enough of. So, try to include potassium-rich foods to your diet. The best sources of potassium you can include in your diet are peas, apricots, cantaloupes, bananas, mushrooms, potatoes, sweet potatoes, and cucumbers.

Vitamin K

It has been getting a lot of attention lately. Vitamin K helps in controlling the protein that is responsible for rebuilding bones. It also provides protection against fractures and a couple of types of cancers. It is quite important for maintaining the overall cardiovascular health since it prevents the accumulation of calcium in the blood vessels. The primary food sources of this vitamin are green leafy vegetables, broccoli, fermented cheeses, and soy products.

Vitamin C

It is responsible for promoting the health of muscles, ligaments, tendons, bones, skin, gums, and cell membranes as well. If you have ever had any problems with your bone strengths or your gums, then you must increase your intake of this vitamin.

Vitamin B-12

It is not quite popular, but this doesn't mean that it isn't important. Vitamin B-12 is essential for maintaining the regular activity that takes place in the nerves in the body. A deficiency in this vitamin causes anemia. Anemia is a condition that is caused when there is depletion in the number of red blood cells present in the body. It is a part of the B-complex vitamin group, and it is essential for maintaining your overall metabolism and energy levels. B-12 is present in meat, salmon, tuna, eggs, and cheese. There aren't many vegetarian or vegan sources of this vitamin. If you follow a vegan or a vegetarian diet, then it is important that you start taking supplements for this vitamin. A lack of this particular vitamin can cause fatigue and shortness of breath.

Vitamin E

It is perhaps the most commonly misunderstood vitamin there is. Just like with the rest of the vitamins, it is important to make sure that you receive this vitamin in a balanced manner. Vitamin is a fat-soluble vitamin, and therefore, it will stay in your system for longer than the water-soluble vitamins. It is present in a vast array of products; therefore, it is quite important that you keep track of your intake of vitamin E. It is an antioxidant and helps in reducing the risk of cardiac diseases and certain types of cancers. It is frequently used in anti-aging treatments and for treating sunburn as well. The best sources of this vitamin are nuts, seeds, and whole grains. There are plenty of vitamin E supplements that you can incorporate into your regular diet.

Magnesium

Another important electrolyte your body needs is magnesium, and a lot of people have a magnesium deficiency without even realizing it. Magnesium helps in the firing of neurons, with digestion, muscle contractions and facilitates heartbeat too. If you have ever experienced a muscle cramp or spasm, it can be due to a magnesium deficiency. So, include magnesium-rich foods or a supplement to your diet.

Before you decide to take any supplements, you must consult a doctor and only then add the necessary supplements to your diet.

Vitamin A

If you were ever fitted for glasses, then you might recollect your doctor mentioning Vitamin A. Vitamin A is responsible for maintaining your vision. Animal liver, free range eggs, and milk are good sources of vitamin A. Include vegetables rich in beta-carotene like spinach, carrots, and cabbage into your daily diet. Using supplements for this vitamin is a good idea because the tolerance level for Vitamin A is quite high. If you have any issues with your eyesight, then you must consider increasing your intake of Vitamin A. A balanced diet must help in preventing the buildup of toxicity in the body.

Chapter 3 – Benefits of the Eat-Stop-Eat Protocol

Why should you consider the Eat-Stop-Eat protocol? It's because more than just healthy weight loss, you may enjoy other potential health benefits. You may be able to lose weight and improve your general health too. Let's take a look at some of the reported health benefits.

Improved Gene, Cells, and Hormonal Functions

Several things occur inside the body when food isn't available for an extended period of time. One of them is initiation of crucial processes that repair damaged cells. Another is changes in hormonal levels that makes it easier for the body to access and burn body fat as energy.

In particular, the body undergoes several changes when in a fasted state such as:

- Insulin levels in the bloodstream plummet to the point where burning fat for energy becomes possible;
- Human growth hormone levels in the bloodstream can spike up to 5 times the normal, which can lead to muscle-building, fat-burning, and other beneficial events in the body;
- Triggering of crucial cell repair processes like flushing out waste from cells; and
- Improvement in terms of genes and molecules related to disease protection and longevity.

Basically, your human growth hormone levels spike and your insulin levels drop when your body is in a fasted state. Such a state also helps you improve your genes and repair damaged cells.

Lower Risks of Type-2 Diabetes

Over the last decade or two, so many people have become diabetic, making diabetes one of the most prevalent life-threatening conditions in the United States. This is because diabetes causes other major health conditions that can potentially be fatal unless managed correctly.

High blood sugar levels are the primary characteristic of diabetes. There are 2 reasons for this: either the pancreas isn't able to produce enough insulin anymore, if any, or the body has become insulin resistant already. The body's inability to produce enough insulin is something that can no longer be remedied but insulin resistance can be lowered in order to lower blood sugar levels and minimize risks of Type-2 or adult onset diabetes.

One of the most interesting finding on intermittent fasting, in general, is that it can be very helpful in significantly reduce insulin resistance and consequently, help reduce blood sugar levels. In clinical studies done on actual people concerning intermittent fasting, blood sugar levels dropped from 3% to 6% and fasting insulin levels dropped from 20% to 31%. And in one particular animal study on diabetes, intermittent fasting has also been shown to reduce risks of kidney damage, which is one of the most serious side effects of diabetes.

What's the implication? Intermittent fasting – such as the Eat-Stop-Eat protocol – can be helpful in reducing risks of Type-2 diabetes. However, this may be more applicable to men because, in one study of diabetic women, a 22-day particular intermittent fasting method actually led to increased blood sugar levels in women.

Lower Oxidative Stress and Inflammation

One of the most potent health killers is oxidative stress. Among other things, it can lead to premature aging and serious chronic conditions. Oxidative stress is characterized by production of unstable molecules – a.k.a. Free radicals – that damage other important molecules like protein and DNA.

Some studies have shown that fasting intermittently, such as when implementing the Eat-Stop-Eat protocol, can improve the human body's ability to fight oxidative stress. Also, studies have shown that intermittent fasting can also be helpful in combatting inflammation in the body, which is another factor in many chronic ailments.

A Healthier Heart

At the time of this writing, heart problems are the number 1 cause of deaths worldwide. And when it comes to risks of heart problems, there are several health markers – a.k.a. Risk factors – that are linked to such risks. Intermittent fasting has been shown in several studies to improve several risk factors for heart problems like:

- Blood pressure;
- Blood sugar levels;
- Inflammation;
- Total and bad (LDL) cholesterol levels; and
- Triglycerides.

The only limitation to the studies that have noted these results is that most of them were conducted on animals.

As such, more human studies must be conducted to reinforce these observed benefits of intermittent fasting.

Improved Cellular Repair

Fasting initiates a process called autophagy, i.e., removal of waste from the cells. Part of this waste-removal process is breaking down dysfunctional proteins in the body that build up in cells over time and metabolizing them. An increase in the body's autophagic process can help reduce risks of certain serious medical conditions like Alzheimer's disease and cancer. Hence, intermittent fasting, like the Eat-Stop-Eat method, can help reduce risks of specific sicknesses by removing more wastes from the body's cells via autophagy.

Lower Risks of Cancers

Fasting has been linked to several metabolic benefits that can lower one's risks of cancer. But because most of the studies that found the cancer risk-lowering benefits of fasting were done on animals, studies on humans need to be done to strongly establish lower cancer risks with intermittent fasting. However, there are studies on human cancer patients that showed fasting's ability to significantly reduce the side effects of chemotherapy.

Healthier Brain

Often times, things that benefit the body also benefit the brain. Another benefit associated with intermittent fasting is improvement of different metabolism-related things that may be considered crucial for brain health. These include lower blood sugar levels, lower insulin resistance, reduced inflammation, and less oxidative stress.

In several rat studies, intermittent fasting has been shown to help increase new nerve cell growth, which can be very beneficial for brain health and performance. I.F. was also shown to help raise BDNF, a.k.a. brain-derived neurotrophic factor, levels in the brain. When there's not enough BDNF, the risks of brain problems like depression are much higher. In other animal studies, intermittent fasting was also shown to be beneficial when it comes to protecting a person's brain from serious injuries due to strokes.

Lower Risk of Alzheimer's

All over the world, the most prevalent neuro-degenerative disease is Alzheimer's disease. The sad part about this is Alzheimer's – as of now – is an incurable condition. So the saying "An ounce of medicine is better than a pound of cure" isn't applicable because there is no cure yet. That means prevention is the only means available to win the fight against it.

Studies on rats showed that when it comes to the onset of this leading neurodegenerative disease, intermittent fasting can help delay it. Same studies also showed that intermittent fasting can help reduce the severity of Alzheimer's. Other animal studies have also shown that intermittent fasting may help protect versus other similar conditions like Huntington's and Parkinson's diseases.

Several case reports also showed that short, daily fasts helped 9 of 10 Alzheimer's patients substantially improve symptoms associated with the condition when included as part of a lifestyle intervention program. But considering most of the studies on intermittent fasting and neurodegenerative diseases were done on animals, more human studies are needed to make an even stronger case for this potentially beneficial effect of intermittent fasting.

Longevity

Given some of the major health benefits one may experience through intermittent fasting, it goes without saying that intermittent fasting may contribute to a generally healthier and longer life.

Chapter 4 – Possible Challenges with Intermittent Fasting

Nothing in the world is perfect. That being said, the Eat-Stop-Eat protocol has its share of potential challenges or negative side effects. These include the following:

Impaired Physical Performance

Particularly during your fasting moments, intermittent fasting may reduce your physical strength as a result of lack of calories from food. This is because energy from food is the easiest to process or access for physical performance compared to body fat. Relying on body fat for energy when it comes to situations where optimal physical performance is crucial, such as sports competitions or when working out, may cause you to perform below optimal levels.

And when you're working out, sub-optimal efforts can keep you from optimizing your body's ability to produce human growth hormone and replenish your glycogen stores immediately after working out. When this happens, your risks of muscle catabolism become high. That's why it's crucial that you synchronize the time of your exercise/workouts with your eating window. That will increase your chances of optimal efforts in the gym and reduce your risks of muscle catabolism.

Potential Eating Disorders

Despite lack of documented studies, dieticians can attest that it is possible to develop eating disorders when fasting intermittently. In particular, many intermittent fasters tend to overcompensate during their eating windows to the point that they were regularly over-eating or worse, binge-eating as they break their fasts. And often times, this happens with unhealthy foods that are highly processed and high in refined sugars and trans fats, which are 2 of the deadliest ingredients in the world found in many commercially available processed foods.

That's why if you're at risk of or are already suffering from an eating disorder, it's best to stay off intermittent fasting. You might aggravate your condition or cause yourself to acquire an eating disorder if fast regularly.

Sterility

Without a shadow of doubt, reproductive health is highly dependent on getting the right nutrients at the right amounts, i.e., adequate calories. An example of this is amenorrhea, which refers to the loss or cessation of a woman's menstrual cycle. This condition has been linked to low body weight and not eating enough.

The exact reasons for this relationship aren't strongly established because human I.F. trials weren't large enough to make certain conclusions. But in one study on female rats, intermittent fasting was shown to obstruct the subjects' fertility.

Sustainability

Regardless of what the staunchest I.F. fanatic says, fasting isn't the norm. Humans are wired to eat so when given opportunities to do so, people would grab them. The only reason why fasting frequently was "natural" thousands of years ago was because of lack of food, which our early ancestors had no control over. In short, they "fasted" against their will.

That being said, it may not be realistic for majority of the human race to fast intermittently for the rest of their lives. Yes, it's possible for some people with extreme levels of self-control and self-discipline to sustain I.F. over the long haul, but they're the exceptions rather than the norm. It's no different from the fact that millions of people all over the world play basketball but only a handful can ever make a serious living out of it regardless of how hard they work at their games.

Now, it doesn't mean you shouldn't fast intermittently. What I'm saying is that it can be very challenging to sustain it over the long haul and if you set your eyes on the long term from the get-go, you might get very disappointed and quit early. The key to making I.F. work for you is to take baby steps. What does that look like?

In terms of doing the Eat-Stop-Eat protocol for example, instead of starting your first fasting days with a full 24-hour fast, start by delaying your breakfast as long as you possibly can. Why?

Believe it or not, you're already fasting intermittently without you knowing it. You do this when you sleep at night, assuming you don't wake up for midnight snacks. So if you get an average of 8 hours of nightly sleep, this means you're already fasting 8 hours every day.

When you delay eating breakfast, you add to that number of hours you fasted overnight. That's why it's more realistic to start this way, e.g., eating an hour or two after waking up. Then gradually move up your breakfast until it becomes brunch and over the next few weeks or months, delay it further until you're able to fast for at least 20 hours, as Brad Pilon suggests.

The reason why many aren't able to sustain it is because they go all gung-ho when they start fasting intermittently, not thinking that fasting is serious business. They get discouraged when they aren't able to sustain their fast long enough to complete it and they drop it altogether. By starting with baby steps and gradually increasing those steps, you'll have a much higher shot at being able to sustain your I.F. protocol long enough to experience its weight loss and other health benefits.

Hypoglycemia

Intermittent fasting results in lower blood sugar levels. But for diabetics, this may not be beneficial. They can't afford to go hungry for extended periods of time because otherwise, their blood sugar levels may drop so low to the point of hypoglycemia. While low blood sugar is generally good, very low blood sugar levels – especially for diabetics – aren't.

So, you should ditch the idea of fasting intermittently if you have diabetes or are already pre-diabetic. Or if you really want to do the Eat-Stop-Eat or other I.F. protocols, consult with your doctor first.

Other Possible Side Effects

Other minor side effects – especially at the beginning – may include:

- Acne;
- Brain fog;

- Caffeine addiction, which may lead to insomnia;
- Constipation;
- Feeling bloated;
- Headaches;
- Heartburn;
- Loose bowel movement;
- Low energy;
- Mood swings; and
- Stronger-than-usual hunger pangs.

Reducing Potential Side Effects

Many of the potential side-effects can be easy to reduce or address. Some of the practical ways by which you can do so include:

- Drink lots of water or calorie-free liquids and during your eating windows, eat foods with high dietary fiber content or supplement with psyllium fiber. If constipation persists, stop fasting and see your doctor.
- Include soluble fiber in what you eat during your eating windows or take mild laxative to address bloating during your I.F..
- Minimize consumption of acid blockers and fatty food to stop heartburn, which normally happens at the beginning of an I.F. If you feel the need to take acid blockers, check with your doctor about which to get and inform him that you're doing I.F.
- Minimize consumption of high-fat and high-sugar foods on your eating days to minimize or stop acne.

Myths About 5:2 Diet

Eating frequently is better for your metabolism

It is nothing but a misconception that you need to keep frequently snacking to improve your metabolism. If you keep eating frequently, you will only be providing your body with a constant source of glucose and will prevent your body from burning any internal fat. Whenever you eat something, your body only uses a small portion of that food as energy and the rest is stored as fat for later use. When you keep eating, you are merely increasing the reserves of fat in the body. So, you need to reduce your calorie intake and give your body a break, if you want it to burn the energy stored within. Your body needs a little energy to digest and absorb the food you consume. About 10% of the calories you consume go toward this, and it is referred to as the thermic effect of food. So, if you consume 2000 calories, the thermic effect of food is 200 calories. Regardless of whether you consume these calories at once or in three meals, the thermic effect stays the same. Therefore, it is safe to say that your body's metabolism doesn't slow down when you limit your calorie intake.

Causes nutrient deficiencies

In the previous section, there was a list of nutrients that your body needs. As long as you ensure that the food you consume has all the necessary nutrients, you don't have to worry about nutrient deficiencies. Consuming healthy and well-balanced meals while following the 5:2 diet protocol will ensure your body gets all the nutrients it needs. The trouble starts when you don't eat nutrient-dense foods and instead munch on unhealthy foods. Yes, you do need to adhere to the calorie restriction. However, it doesn't mean that you eat a packet of chips on the day of the fast and expect the diet to work. Doing this might lead to weight loss, but it will certainly deprive your body of the essential nutrients.

Loss of muscle mass

Protein catabolism occurs when there is a depletion of liver glycogen, and it leads to loss of muscle mass. Simply put, at such a stage, your body will start to cannibalize its muscle tissue, and the amino acids present within are converted into glucose to support your body. When your body starts running out of these essential amino acids, it looks for other sources of amino acids. If you deprive your body of glucose for over 28 hours, only then will your body start digesting its muscles. Up until then, you have nothing to worry about. While following the 5:2 diet, you will merely need to reduce your calorie intake, so you don't have to worry about losing muscle mass. In fact, by following this diet and combining it with the necessary exercises, you can build lean muscle.

Eating disorders

If you stick to your diet and consume wholesome meals, you don't have to worry about developing any eating disorders. If you want to maintain a healthy relationship with food, then you must consume healthy meals and skimp on the necessary nutrients. However, if you ever suffered from an eating disorder in the past, are recovering from one or are suffering from an eating disorder, then don't diet unless your doctor thinks it is safe for you.

Causes fertility troubles for women

Women tend to have different nutrient requirements than men. Some people tend to believe that intermittent fasting causes fertility issues for women. Well, this is nothing more than a misconception. Unless you are pregnant or lactating, then this diet is safe for a healthy adult to follow. While following this diet, you must ensure that you are carefully following the protocols mentioned and fast responsibly.

Chapter 5 – Exercise: Rev Up Your Weight Loss Results

The Eat-Stop-Eat can help you lose excess body fat and body weight. But as with any serious weight loss effort, combining a healthy and sensible fat-loss diet can help speed up the process. This is because it can help prevent or even speed up your metabolism and burn more body fat in the process. Resistance training exercises can help you preserve or even increase muscle mass, which is very important for a healthy metabolism.

Personally, I find that people who lose weight through a combination of diet and exercise tend to look better than people who lost weight through dieting alone. Those who include exercise in their weight loss strategy end up looking fitter and stronger compared to those that only diet. Hence, you should seriously consider incorporating regular exercise with the Eat-Stop-Eat protocol.

If you decide to incorporate regular exercise into your Eat-Stop-Eat, here are some practical tips for optimizing the benefits of regular exercise while fasting intermittently.

Optimal Timing

According to nutrition expert Christopher Shuff, you should ask yourself whether you should schedule your workouts before, within, or after your eating windows. To help you choose which time is the best time, you must think about what your goal is for exercising during your I.F.

If your primary goal is to burn as much body fat as possible, then try working out in a fasted state, i.e., 1 ½ hours before your eating window or at least 3 hours the window is optimal. Being in a fasted state will force your body to tap your glycogen and eventually, your body fat stores for energy during exercise. This optimizes fat-burning, but the trade-off is reduced physical performance, i.e., less weight lifted or lower exercise intensity.

But if your primary goal is optimal performance or strength and muscle building, you should schedule your workouts during your eating windows. Why? It's because you'll need all the easily accessible energy you can get to go all out on your workout sessions.

Another thing to consider is your own physical fitness level. If you're already used to performing physical exercises at a relatively high level even if you haven't eaten within 3 to 4 hours prior, i.e., a fasted state, then working out during your fasting days or before your eating window can be your best option for fat-burning. If you're not, then you'd be better off working out during your eating days.

Kinds of Workouts

Lynda Lippin, who's a certified personal trainer, says being cognizant of the calories or macronutrients you consumed the day prior to working out and those that you eat after. She says that if you want to do strength training exercises, you must make sure you get enough carbohydrates the day before and on the day of the workout itself. But if you plan to do cardio or high intensity interval workouts (HIIT), you can schedule it on days when you eat less carbohydrates.

Within the context of the Eat-Stop-Eat protocol and what Lippin said, you may be better off lifting weights during your eating days and doing steady state cardio or HIIT exercises during your fasting days for optimal fat-burning.

Post-Workout Nutrition

As mentioned earlier, scheduling your weight lifting or resistance training workouts during your regular eating days is optimal for fat-burning. This is because aside from having enough fuel to power your muscles for the heavy workload ahead, it also provides your muscles with much needed nutrients to avoid muscle catabolism. Remember, muscle catabolism can substantially slow down your metabolism. Hence, the need to avoid at all costs.

A good post-workout nutrition guide is to consume a good amount of carbohydrates, particularly starchy carbohydrates with around 20 grams of good quality protein after at least 1 hour. Why that long? According to top fitness and nutrition expert Shaun Hadsall of the Over 40 Ab Solution program, waiting for at least an hour after you end your exercise allows you to "ride" your body's fat-burning wave and burn more fat before you nourish your muscles with much-needed protein and glycogen.

Pre-Workout Nutrition

For optimal physical performance during your weight-lifting sessions, you'll need to ensure your body's glycogen stores are filled up. Doing so will ensure you have enough fuel to power through a very grueling weight-lifting session.

Hydration and Electrolyte Levels

When exercising, always keep a bottle of water close by so you can continually stay hydrated regardless if lifting weights at the gym on your eating days or doing steady state cardio on your fasting days. Ideally, drink between 17 to 20 ounces of water 2 to 3 hours prior to working out or doing steady state cardio and another 8 ounces 30 minutes prior. During exercise, drink between 7 and 10 ounces every 10 to 20 minutes. Post exercise drink another 8 ounces within 30 minutes.

If you're particular about maintaining good electrolyte levels, consider drinking fresh, plain coconut water. It's high in electrolytes but, unlike sports drinks like Gatorade, it is low in sugar and total calories, which makes it perfect for your fat-burning goals.

Intensity and Duration

When exercising during your fasting days, it's best to keep exercise duration and intensity between low to medium only. This is because you aren't getting any calories that day, which will make you significantly less strong with shorter stamina. If you push it to the hilt, you may feel dizzy or worse, faint from sheer exhaustion. That's why the best workout for your fasting days – should you decide to exercise – is low to medium intensity steady state cardio for up to 30 minutes maximum. Examples of low to moderate steady state cardio include brisk walking on the road or on a treadmill, leisurely biking around the neighborhood on relatively level ground, and stationary biking.

Pay Attention to Your Body

Your fasting day isn't the time to go all gung-ho by dismissing what your body's telling you, especially if it's telling you how bad it already feels. If you feel dizzy or weak, stop exercising. Chances are high that you're either dehydrated, low in blood sugar, or both. Drink lots of water and rest. If you still feel dizzy from hunger, don't be a martyr and insist on continuing your fast for that day. Ditch that day's fast, drink an electrolyte-rich drink and eat a healthy meal to normalize your blood sugar levels too. Sports drinks are okay in this situation, given your low electrolyte and blood sugar levels. Just learn your lesson and keep your cardio session levels to moderate at most and for 30 minutes maximum only on your succeeding fasting days.

Exercising on the Eat-Stop-Eat Protocol

If you're wondering how a good exercise program may look like on the Eat-Stop-Eat program, first thing you'll need to consider is getting enough cardiovascular exercise. This type of exercise can help make your heart stronger along with other muscles in your body. If you plan to do cardio work on your fasting days, keep it at moderate intensity at most and 30 minutes at the longest. If you plan to do it on your eating days, you can go for a high intensity and/or longer duration (up to 45 minutes maximum) cardio workout. Do cardio exercises 2 to 3 times weekly.

Second, incorporate strength and resistance training into your exercise regimen. Why? As mentioned earlier, it can help tone your muscles, so you don't look frail and gaunt. Not only that, it can help you minimize muscle catabolism and it can raise your resting metabolism for longer periods of time after exercising compared to cardio exercises. This means you get to burn more body fat even while at rest! This is called the "afterburn" effect.

There are 2 kinds of resistance or weight-lifting exercises: compound and isolation. Compound exercises – also referred to as multi-joint exercises – are those that involve multiple muscle groups at a time. Isolation exercises – also known as single-joint exercises – involve only a single muscle group, which results in just moving a single joint in the body.

If you want to optimize strength building and fat burning, prioritize compound exercises over isolation ones. Why? It's because by virtue of using more muscle groups, you burn more calories and consequently, body fat! Talk about getting more fat-burning bang for your exercise buck!

Three of the best compound weight-lifting exercises you can do are barbell squats, barbell or dumbbell deadlifts, and barbell or dumbbell bench presses. Squats involve the entire leg muscle group (the biggest muscle group in the body), the lower back and abdominal muscles (the core muscles) for stabilization, and shoulders and upper back muscles for balancing the barbell. So, you practically work out your entire body (except for chest and arms) with just one exercise!

The next best compound exercise is the deadlift. This exercise primarily works on your lower back and hamstrings, i.e., the muscle below your butt and above the back of your knees. For stabilization, it also involves your abdominal muscles, your thighs, your calves, your forearms (for holding the barbell or dumbbell) and biceps. The heavier the weight you hoist, the more calories and body fat you can burn. You also get stronger and more muscular, too.

The bench press primarily works out your chest and triceps muscles, but for stabilization, it also involves your shoulders and your abdominal muscles.

Other compound lifting exercises worth doing are:

- Barbell rows;
- Bodyweight or weighted dips;
- Chin ups (bodyweight or weighted);
- Clean presses;
- Dumbbell or barbell lunges;
- Incline bench presses;
- Standing barbell curls; and
- Standing military presses.

Isolation exercises are good exercises for finishing off your workouts and creating good detail in your muscles if you're the type who wants to look buffed and toned. It also helps you burn additional calories. However, these should only be optional exercises, i.e., you should only do them when you have extra time and energy after performing compound exercises. Examples of isolation exercises include:

- Calf raises;
- Crunches;
- Leg curls;
- Leg extensions;
- Seated dumbbell curls;
- Side laterals;
- Single-arm overhead dumbbell triceps extensions;
- Sit-ups; and
- Wrist curls.

Muscle Recovery

Before you work out again, you should ensure that your muscles are fully rested and recovered from the previous one. Doing so can help lower your risks of injuries, burnout, and fatigue. So, what's a good guideline for this?

Your muscles need at least 48 hours of rest and recovery before being worked out again for optimal performance and reduced risks of injuries. If you worked out your chest on Monday afternoon, the earliest you should be doing it again is Wednesday afternoon.

What if you perform a whole-body routine, i.e., you work out all the major muscle groups in one workout? An optimal way to go about this is to do your steady state cardio in between gym days. You may even take advantage of this to schedule your fasting days in between your weight-lifting days.

Supplementation

When you're fasting, you're not getting enough calories for 2 of the 7 days of the week. This can result in some nutritional deficiencies and can weaken your immune system. That's why it's important to take multivitamins and other nutrients in supplemental form such as protein, etc.

Sleep

Regardless of your stand on sleep, you'll need to get adequate amounts of it more so if you're fasting intermittently. And more than just the amount, you'll need quality sleep, too. If you sleep for 10 hours a night, but your sleep is shallow, you'll feel like you only get 3 hours of sleep nightly. So, the key is both quality and duration. The deeper your sleep, the lesser the hours.

If you're the type of person who sleeps poorly, both in terms of duration and quality, here are 3 hacks you can try individually or collectively. Personally, I use them collectively and the results are very, very good!

Deep Sleep Hack #1: Sleep Tonic

I picked this up from one of Tim Ferriss' podcasts where he shared the sleep tonic recipe he swears by for deep sleep. It consists of:

- 1 cup warm water;
- 1 tablespoon of real honey; and
- 2 tablespoons of apple cider vinegar, preferably Bragg's.

Just mix the 3 and drink before bedtime. Don't ask me – or Tim Ferriss – how it works. It just does. Though you might want to skip this if you have hyperacidity issues.

Deep Sleep Hack #2: Synchronize with Your Sleep Cycle

Recent scientific studies have discovered that on average, humans sleep in 90-minute cycles. Each cycle consists of 5 sleep stages, the deepest of which is stage 4. If you want to have an easier time waking up in the morning and feeling more alert and rested, you should wake up at a time that coincides with the end of a 90-minute sleep cycle.

Let's say you sleep at 9:00 pm. The most optimal times for you to wake up based on 90-minute cycles are:

- End of sleep cycle #1: 10:45 pm (1 hour and 45 minutes of sleep)
- End of sleep cycle #2: 12:15 am (3 hours and 15 minutes of sleep)
- End of sleep cycle #3: 1:45 am (4 hours and 45 minutes of sleep)
- End of sleep cycle #4: 3:15 am (6 hours and 15 minutes of sleep)
- End of sleep cycle #5: 4:45 am (7 hours and 45 minutes of sleep)
- End of sleep cycle # 6: 6:15 am (9 hours and 15 minutes of sleep)

If you wake up in the middle of a sleep cycle, especially during stage 4 (the deepest stage), you will have a very hard time waking up and chances are, you'll feel sluggish for most part of the morning.

Two of the best apps are Sleep Cycle Alarm Clock (iPhone) and Sleep Time (for Android). These apps will tell you what times you should wake up if you sleep now or what time you should sleep if you want to wake up at a certain time.

Deep Sleep Hack #3: Binaural Beats

These refer to sounds that result from combining two slightly different sound frequencies. The resulting sounds are perceived by its listeners as single tone frequencies.

The main idea behind binaural beats is that audibly exposing the brain to 2 different frequencies simultaneously, one frequency for each ear, makes it perceive one tone to which it will tune in. Scientific studies have shown that listening to a low-frequency tone slows down brainwave activity to the point where a person can feel more relaxed, less anxious, and have a much easier time falling into and staying in deep sleep.

The best way to use binaural beats for sleep is to listen to delta wave binaural beats (0.1 to 4 Hz frequencies) using stereo earphones. The stereo earphones are necessary because as mentioned earlier, the single tone is created by 2 different frequencies, each played in one ear. Unless played separately in each ear, the binaural beat frequencies won't be perceived by the brain.

Chapter 6 – Practical Tips for Successful Fasting

As we end this book, I want to give you some practical ways to maximize your chances of succeeding with intermittent fasting. Some of them may even apply to other areas of your life, particularly with starting something new and challenging that you'll need to sustain over a significant amount of time.

A Clear and Compelling Reason

Why do you want to fast intermittently using the Eat-Stop-Eat diet? Unless you're clear about it and unless it's compelling, I'm afraid your chances of succeeding are low. Why?

With a clear and compelling reason, you'll have enough motivation to stay the course even when the going gets really tough. If your reason for doing the Eat-Stop-Eat is shallow or flimsy, your chances of quitting after your 1st or 2nd 24-hour fasting day will be very, very high.

While losing weight and looking/feeling great are valid reasons for doing the Eat-Stop-Eat protocol, those aren't very compelling reasons. To clarify your compelling reason for doing the protocol, ask "Why" until it's no longer possible to ask the question.

For example, you want to lose weight, so you decide to get into the Eat-Stop-Eat protocol. Why do you want to lose weight? If that's your end goal, I'm sorry, but it will not get you through when things get tough in the Eat-Stop-

Eat diet. But if the reason you want to lose weight is to bring your health risks down and be as healthy as you can be, ask yourself why health is that important to you? Some sensible answers include:

- Because you want to see your children grow up to be adults and have their own children too;
- Because you don't want your wife to get widowed early and be lonely for the rest of her life; and
- Because you don't want to die a slow and painful death due to debilitating diseases like cancer, diabetes, or heart problems.

Having clear and compelling reasons like these will make you feel that the challenges and sacrifices you'll need to make on the Eat-Stop-Eat protocol will be worth it. And when you feel that way, you can power through the difficult stages of the protocol.

Feed Before the Fast

I'm not talking about eating food but feeding your mind prior to fasting so you can be in the right mindset and be optimally prepared when you finally take action. What does feeding the mind prior to the actual implementation of the Eat-Stop-Eat protocol look like? Here are some ideas:

- Read books, blogs, or articles and watch vlogs about the Eat-Stop-Eat method; and
- If you know people who have successfully accomplished their weight and health goals via the protocol or intermittent fasting in general, reach out to them so you can have reasonable expectations about your up-and-coming Eat-Stop-Eat journey.

By getting enough experiential information about Eat-Stop-Eat, you can prepare yourself well.

Build Up Your Fasting Endurance

One of the reasons why many people drop out of the intermittent fasting game, in general, is hitting the ground running at full throttle. By this, I mean they try to fast for 20 to 24 hours immediately without giving their bodies and minds the chance to adjust to such a rigorous practice. Going without food for 20 to 24 hours straight isn't something to be taken lightly.

Can you imagine Usain Bolt, the fastest man in sprinting history, sprinting at maximum speed directly after getting up from bed in the morning? Stupid, right? He won't be able to run at top speed straight from waking up and worse, he can tear a muscle or ligament by going all out without the benefit of warming up and limbering his leg muscles.

It's the same with intermittent fasting, particularly for protocols like the Eat-Stop-Eat, which require 24-hour fasts. It's not something ordinary humans can do. Hence, it can be very, very hard or even impossible for a beginner to successfully complete a 24-hour fast straight out of the gate.

A very good starting point is your average nightly sleeping hours. Let's say you sleep an average of 8 hours nightly. That's already 8 hours of fasting. If you take breakfast within 30 minutes upon waking up and if you eat your last meal of the day 1 hour before bed, it means you're already fasting for 9 ½ hours nightly on average. Let that be your baseline.

Start by adding an hour or two to your baseline by delaying your breakfast. If you delay your breakfast by an hour, or 1 ½ hours after waking up, you extend your fasting endurance to 10 ½ hours already. If you normally skip breakfast and go straight to lunch, then you're already fasting for over 12 hours every day.

Gradually delay your first meal of the day by 1 hour every week or two or eat your last meal 1 hour earlier than you normally would every week or two. By doing that, you can gradually build up your fasting endurance.

Plan Your Fasting Days

Because you'll have no access to calories on your fasting days, it's best to schedule them on your least physically but non-consecutive busy days, especially if you'll schedule your steady state cardio exercises on those days. But if you're the type of person who finds it easier to diet during your busiest days of the week because your mind's preoccupied with a lot of things, you can schedule it on 2 of your busiest days of the week.

Work on Your Mental Barriers

Most of the concerns about fasting are mental, except in situations when a person is experiencing real physiological and physical danger during a very severe fast. Many people have already disqualified themselves from fasting even before giving it a shot by thinking, "I'm not built for it" or "I can't control my appetite." In other words, many people aren't able to fast intermittently simply because they've already decided in their minds that they can't do it.

Here's something to – pardon the pun – chew on as you contemplate on the Eat-Stop-Eat protocol: People of average weight can live without food for up to 40 days. That's 40 frickin' days! With the Eat-Stop-Eat, you'll only need to fast 2 days a week. And it's not even 2 straight days because you should fast on 2 non-consecutive days.

Many times, the hunger that we feel are either mental or a simple case of dehydration, in which case drinking a glass or two of water is enough to quell hunger pangs. Unless you have a pre-existing medical condition that can be aggravated by fasting regularly, there's very little reason to believe that you can't succeed at intermittent fasting.

When you think about it, physical barriers are easier to dismantle or breakthrough than mental ones. And one of the best ways to gradually break down mental barriers to intermittent fasting is by increasing one's knowledge about it. In particular, a highly recommended resource is the book Eat-Stop-Eat by no less than the man himself, Brad Pilon.

Don't Broadcast It

Next, to your mental barriers, the next biggest obstacles are the people around you, particularly their negative reactions and potentially discouraging words. This shouldn't be a surprise, especially from your family members. They will probably be critical of your Eat-Stop-Eating plans because of 2 things: genuine concern for you and ignorance of intermittent fasting. Hence, you must do your best to not let other people know what you're doing unless they've already done intermittent fasting or are knowledgeable about its health-related benefits.

Keep Hunger at Bay

If you are following the 5:2 diet, then you will be restricting your calorie intake on the fast days. One of the major reasons why a lot of dieters give up on their diets is because of hunger. If you learn to keep your hunger pangs at bay, it will become easier to stick to the diet. Also, by understanding your hunger cues, you can differentiate between real and psychological hunger. Instead of eating whenever you think you are hungry, you will learn to eat only when your body needs to eat. Hunger pangs are quite common during the first couple of weeks of fasting when your body is getting used to the calorie restriction. In this section, you will learn about the different tips you can follow to keep hunger pangs at bay.

You must ensure that you are keeping your body hydrated always. Dehydration can make you feel quite tired and even cause a headache. Also, the best way to curb hunger is by drinking water. Whenever you experience a hunger pang, drink a glass of water, give yourself twenty minutes, and the hunger pang will pass. At times, you might think you are hungry, but it might just be thirst. So, staying hydrated while fasting will improve your overall health and help you control your hunger too.

Whenever a hunger pang strikes you, it can be difficult to focus on anything other than the hunger pangs. The best thing to do at such times is to remind yourself of the reasons why you started the diet. You might want to improve your overall health or might want to lose weight. Regardless of your reasons for dieting, it is a good idea to remind yourself of the same. You can make a list of all the reasons why you want to diet and glance at the list whenever you feel like giving in to any unhealthy cravings.

Coffee is one of the best ways to curb hunger pangs. If you are used to drinking coffee as soon as you wake up in the morning, then it will give you the necessary energy to keep going until lunchtime. You can substitute coffee with tea too. However, you cannot add any milk or sugar to these beverages since it will only increase your calorie intake. Try to stick to herbal teas and black coffee.

You can distract yourself from thinking about food by focusing on activities you like or even your work. When you occupy yourself with work, you will not have the time to think about food or hunger. Have there been times when you were so engrossed with the work that you forgot to eat? Well, you will essentially be trying to recreate this scenario. All protocols of intermittent fasting tend to free up a lot of your time, and you can use this time to work on things you love. If you have a hobby you enjoy, then go ahead and spend some time on it. By staying productive, you can prevent your mind from thinking about food.

Focusing on your dental hygiene is another way to ensure that you complete your fast. Having fresh and minty breath tends to reduce your desire to eat. On the fast days, after you eat a meal or a snack, don't forget to brush your teeth quickly. It is a way to signal your mind that you are done eating. It will not only improve your oral health but will help keep those cravings in check.

Don't take a lot of stress and learn to keep calm. When you are under stress, your body releases cortisol, a stress-inducing hormone that increases your desire to eat. The more stressed you are, the greater will be your desire to eat. Learning to control your stress has other health benefits like stabilizing your blood pressure and improving your ability to sleep. Apart from this, it also helps with better decision making and gives you mental clarity. So, by learning to control stress, it will not only help curb hunger pangs but will improve your overall health too. Try to spend some time outdoors, talk to a friend, spend time with your loved ones, or do anything else that will make you feel calm and relaxed.

Whenever you eat, you must ensure that your meals are rich in protein, fiber, and naturally fatty food. When you consume nutrient-dense foods, it helps you feel fuller for longer. Not just that, but it also provides your body with all the nutrients it needs.

On the days of the fast, make sure that you don't just slouch on your couch all day long. When your mind is idle, it tends to start thinking. So, get on with your day and move around a little. Don't opt for a sedentary lifestyle if you want to be able to stick to this diet.

There is another simple way to curb hunger, and that's by chewing gum. The chewing motion helps trick your mind into thinking you are full and helps keep hunger at bay.

Stay Motivated

At times, it can become rather difficult to stick to the diet. You might be surrounded by plenty of temptations, or you might even feel disheartened. Regardless of the reason, here are three simple tips you can use to ensure that your motivation levels don't falter while dieting.

The first thing you must do is start using the mirror instead of a weighing scale to gauge your progress. When you get started with the diet, stand in front of a full-length mirror and look at all the areas in your body you want to lose weight from. If you want, you can take a picture of yourself. As you continue to follow the diet, there might be times when the diet works, but you cannot see a change in the weighing scales. If that's the case, then use the picture to see the improvement. You might not notice a sudden dip in the scales, but after a couple of weeks, you can see a positive change in your body measurements.

It is also a good idea to start a diet with a partner. You can team up with a friend, family member, colleague, or even your spouse. Going through a diet when you have someone to keep you company makes things easier. Not just that, you will also have a support system in place. You can fast, exercise, shop for groceries, and plan the meals together. Whenever you feel like giving up, you will have someone to help you stay on track and keep going.

You must make it a point to include different foods to your diet. If you keep eating the same items daily, you will certainly get bored. It is quintessential to ensure that your diet doesn't get repetitive or boring. Make a meal plan for all the fasting and non-fasting days, look for healthy recipes online, and stock up your pantry with the necessary ingredients.

Chapter 7 - Breakfast Recipes

Peach, Raspberry and Nuts Smoothie

Serves: 1

Ingredients:

For smoothie:

- ½ cup fresh raspberries
- 1 peach, pitted, sliced
- 1mmedium banana, sliced
- ½ cup low fat yogurt
- 25-30 almonds, soaked in water for a few hours

For topping:

- 2-3 raspberries
- 2 soaked almonds, slivered
- 2-3 peach slices

Directions:

1. Gather all the ingredients for a smoothie and add into a blender.
2. Blend for 30-40 seconds or until smooth.
3. Pour into a tall glass. Add crushed ice if desired.
4. Top with raspberries, almonds and peaches and serve.

Oatmeal Smoothie

Serves: 2

Ingredients:

- ½ cup old fashioned oats or quick oats
- 1 cup unsweetened almond milk
- 1 tablespoon pure maple syrup +extra to garnish
- 1 teaspoon ground cinnamon
- Ice cubes, as required, crushed (optional)
- 2 bananas, sliced, frozen
- 2 tablespoons creamy peanut butter
- 1 teaspoon pure vanilla extract
- ¼ teaspoon kosher salt

Directions:

1. Gather all the ingredients for smoothie. Set aside the ice and add the rest of the ingredients into a blender.
2. Blend for 30-40 seconds or until smooth. Add ice and pulse for a few seconds.
3. Pour into tall glasses and serve.

Acai Smoothie Bowl

Serves: 2

Ingredients:

- 1 large bananas, sliced, frozen
- ¼ cup soy milk
- 7 ounces unsweetened acai berry pulp, frozen

For topping:

- 4 tablespoons granola
- 1 large banana, sliced

Directions:

1. Add banana, acai berry pulp and soy sauce into a blender and blend until thick and smooth.
2. Divide into 2 bowls. Top with banana slices and granola and serve.

Cinnamon Porridge with Grated Pear

Serves: 4

Ingredients:

- 4.5 ounces jumbo porridge oats
- 20 ounces semi-skimmed milk
- Juice of a lemon
- ½ teaspoon ground cinnamon + extra to garnish
- 2 ripe medium pears, peeled, cored, grated

Directions:

1. Add oats, milk and cinnamon into a non-stick saucepan. Place the saucepan over medium heat
2. Stir constantly until thick.
3. Divide into 4 bowls.
4. Top with grated pears. Drizzle lemon juice on top and serve.

Crunchy Banana Yoghurt

Serves: 1

Ingredients:

- 6 ounces fat-free natural Greek yogurt

Toppings: Use any one or more

- 1 teaspoon pumpkin seeds
- 1 teaspoon sesame seeds
- 1 teaspoon sunflower seeds
- Toasted, slivered almonds
- 1 small banana sliced

Directions:

1. Add yogurt into a bowl. Place banana slices on top.
2. Sprinkle the suggested toppings and serve.

Asparagus-Goat Cheese Soufflés

Serves: 3

Ingredients:

- ½ pound asparagus, trimmed
- 1 tablespoon butter
- 1 ½ tablespoons all-purpose flour
- Freshly ground pepper to taste
- Salt to taste
- 4 large egg whites, at room temperature
- 2 large yolks, at room temperature
- A pinch ground nutmeg
- ¾ cup hot non-fat milk

Directions:

1. Place a large pan over high heat. Add water to cover ¼ of the skillet. When it begins to boil, place the asparagus in it and cover the pan partially.
2. Cook until the asparagus is crisp as well as tender. Drain and rinse under cold running water.
3. Dry the asparagus by patting with a kitchen towel.
4. Cut into ½ inch pieces
5. Grease 3 ramekins with cooking spray and place on a rimmed baking sheet.
6. Place rack at the bottom of the oven.
7. Place a saucepan over medium-low heat. Add butter. When butter melts, add flour and stir constantly for a couple of minutes. Remove from heat.
8. Add milk and whisk well. Place the saucepan back over medium-low heat, stirring constantly until thick. Add salt, pepper and nutmeg. Turn off the heat.
9. Add yolks, one at a time and whisk well each time until well incorporated. Spoon the mixture into a bowl.
10. Add whites into another bowl and beat with an electric mixer until frothy.

11. Add salt to taste and beat until soft peaks are formed. Do not overbeat.
12. Add 1/3 of the whites into the bowl of yolks and fold gently. Similarly add the remaining whites and fold gently.
13. Spoon into the ramekins. Fill up to nearly the top.
14. Place the baking sheet along with the ramekins on the rack.
15. Bake in a preheated oven at 375° F for 20 to 25 minutes or until the top is risen and golden brown.

Mushroom Hash with Poached Eggs

Serves: 2

Ingredients:

- 2 teaspoons rapeseed oil
- ½ pound button mushrooms, quartered
- 3-4 fresh tomatoes, chopped
- 2 teaspoons omega seed mix
- 1 large onion, sliced
- ½ tablespoon chopped fresh thyme leaves + extra to garnish
- ½ teaspoon smoked paprika
- 2 large eggs, poached
- Pepper to taste
- Salt to taste

Directions:

1. Place a non-stick pan over medium heat. Add oil. When the oil is heated, add onion and sauté until translucent.
2. Lower the heat and cover with a lid. Cook for 3-4 minutes.
3. Stir in mushrooms and thyme and sauté until tender.
4. Stir in tomatoes and paprika. Cover again and cook until tomatoes are soft.
5. Add seed mix and stir.
6. Divide into 2 plates. Top with poached egg and serve.

Honey Lime Quinoa Fruit Salad

Serves: 2-3

Ingredients:

- ½ cup uncooked quinoa, rinsed
- ½ cup blackberries
- ¾ cup sliced strawberries
- ½ cup blackberries
- ½ cup chopped ripe mango

For honey lime glaze:

- 2 tablespoons honey
- ½ tablespoon chopped basil, to garnish
- 1 tablespoon lime juice

Directions:

1. Cook quinoa following the directions on the package.
2. Cool completely. Fluff with a fork. Transfer into a bowl.
3. Add all the berries and mango and toss well.
4. To make honey lime glaze: Add honey and lime juice into a bowl and stir. Pour over the salad. Toss well.
5. Sprinkle basil on top and serve.

Peanut Butter Banana Overnight Oats

Serves: 2-3

Ingredients:

- 2 cups old fashioned oats
- 2-4 teaspoon agave nectar or honey
- ½ cup creamy peanut butter or almond butter
- 1 large banana, sliced
- 2 tablespoons chia seeds
- 2 cups vanilla soy milk

To serve:

- 1 banana, sliced

Directions:

1. Add banana, peanut butter and soymilk into a blender.
2. Blend for 30-40 seconds or until smooth.
3. Pour into an airtight container.
4. Add honey and stir. Add chia seeds and oats and stir. Cover and refrigerate overnight.
5. Stir and spoon into bowls.
6. Top with banana slices and serve.

Chapter 8 - Salad, Soup and Stew Recipes

Mexican Tempeh Quinoa Salad

Serves: 2

Ingredients:

- ½ cup quinoa
- ½ tablespoon olive oil
- 1 cup water
- 1 small onion, chopped
- 4 ounces tempeh, chopped into bite size pieces
- ½ red bell pepper, diced
- ½ cup salsa
- ½ teaspoon ground cumin
- Salt to taste
- Cayenne pepper to taste
- Pepper to taste
- ½ cup corn, fresh or frozen
- 1 tablespoon chopped fresh cilantro
- ½ avocado, peeled, pitted, diced
- Juice of ½ lime
- ½ can (from a 15 ounces can) black beans, rinsed, drained
- ¼ cup halved cherry tomatoes

Directions:

1. Add quinoa and water into a small pot. Cover the pot and place over high heat.
2. When it begins to boil, lower the heat and simmer until dry. Turn off the heat and set aside.
3. Meanwhile, place a pan over medium heat. Add oil. When the oil is heated, add onion and sauté until translucent.

4. Stir in the tempeh, bell pepper, lime juice, salsa, salt and spices. Cook for 10-12 minutes until tempeh is cooked.
5. Fluff the quinoa with a fork and add into a large glass bowl. Add the tempeh mixture and stir gently.
6. Add rest of the ingredients and toss gently.
7. Serve warm or at room temperature.

Warm Chicken Salad

Serves: 4

Ingredients:

- 4 small chicken breasts, skinless, boneless, halved
- 2 large orange or red bell pepper, deseeded, cut into 1 inch squares
- 3 1/2 ounces watercress, discard hard stalks
- 1 medium cucumber, sliced
- 2 little gem lettuce, leaves separated
- 4 medium tomatoes, chopped
- 2 teaspoons thick balsamic vinegar
- Sea salt to taste
- Freshly ground pepper to taste
- Cooking spray

Directions:

1. Sprinkle salt and pepper over the chicken.
2. Place a large nonstick pan over high heat. Spray with cooking spray.
3. Add chicken and cook until light brown all over. Remove onto your chopping board. Cook in batches if required. Spray the pan in each batch. When cool enough to handle, cut into slices.
4. Spray some oil in the pan. Add bell pepper and cook until slightly charred. Turn off the heat.
5. Divide the lettuce among 4 plates. Divide and place watercress, tomatoes and cucumber over the lettuce.
6. Scatter the cooked bell pepper. Place chicken slices all over. Drizzle balsamic vinegar and lemon juice on top. Sprinkle pepper on top and serve.

Chicken and Broccoli Slaw Salad with Blue Cheese Yogurt Dressing

Serves: 3-4

Ingredients:

<u>For dressing:</u>

- 1 cup plain yogurt
- 2 tablespoons apple cider vinegar
- 2 teaspoons lemon juice
- ¼ cup blue cheese crumbles

<u>For salad:</u>

- 1 green onion, thinly sliced
- 4 ounces grilled or baked chicken breast, shredded or chopped
- 4 cups broccoli slaw

Directions:

1. To make dressing: Whisk together all the ingredients of dressing in a bowl.
2. For salad: Add broccoli slaw in a bowl. Add dressing and stir until well coated.
3. Place chicken breast on top. Garnish with green onion and serve.

Tomato, Cucumber, and Avocado Salad

Serves: 4-6

Ingredients:

- 12 small tomatoes, cut into wedges
- 2 large avocados, pitted, peeled, chopped
- ½ cup chopped basil
- 4 tablespoons olive oil
- 2 English cucumbers, peeled if desired, cut into half-moon slices
- 1 small red onion, thinly sliced
- 6 tablespoons white balsamic vinegar
- Salt to taste
- Pepper to taste

Directions:

1. Add tomatoes, avocado, cucumber and red onions in a large bowl.
2. Pour balsamic vinegar and olive oil over it. Toss well.
3. Sprinkle salt and pepper to taste. Toss well.
4. Garnish with basil and serve.

Wild Rice and Mushroom Soup

Serves: 4

Ingredients:

- ½ pound baby Portobello mushrooms, chopped
- 1 package (6 ounces) long grain wild rice mix
- ¼ cup water
- 1 tablespoon olive oil
- 2 cups low sodium beef broth
- 1 cup heavy cream

Directions:

1. Place a soup pot over medium heat. Add oil. When the oil is heated, add mushrooms and cook until it releases some of its moisture.
2. Stir in the rice along with seasoning mix.
3. Add broth and water and stir.
4. When it begins to boil, lower the heat and cover with a lid. Simmer until wild rice is tender.
5. Stir in cream. Heat thoroughly.
6. Ladle into soup bowls and serve.

Mexican Cabbage Soup

Serves: 4

Ingredients:

- 1 tablespoon extra-virgin olive oil
- 1 medium carrot, chopped
- 1 large onion, chopped
- 1 stalk celery, chopped
- 2 large cloves garlic, minced
- ½ cup chopped green bell pepper or poblano pepper
- 4 cups sliced cabbage
- ½ tablespoon minced chipotle chili in adobo sauce
- ¼ teaspoon ground coriander2 cups water
- Salt to taste
- 1 tablespoon lime juice
- ½ tablespoon tomato paste
- ½ teaspoon ground cumin
- 2 cups vegetable broth or chicken broth
- 1 an (15 ounces) pinto or black beans, rinsed
- ¼ cup chopped cilantro + extra to garnish

To serve:

- Chopped avocado
- ¼ cup crumbled queso fresco
- Plain Greek yogurt

Directions:

1. Place a soup pot over medium heat. Add oil. When the oil is heated, add onion, celery, carrot, bell pepper and garlic and sauté until slightly tender.
2. Stir in the cabbage and cook until slightly soft.
3. Whisk in the tomato paste, cumin, coriander and chipotle chili. Stir constantly for a minute.
4. Stir in broth, water, salt and beans. Cover and lower the heat. Simmer until the vegetables are cooked as per your preference. Turn off the heat.
5. Add cilantro and lime juice and stir.

6. Ladle into soup bowls.
7. Sprinkle cheese and avocado on top. Drizzle yogurt on top and serve.

Paprika & Red Pepper Soup with Pistachio Puree

Serves: 8

Ingredients:

- 4 tablespoons canola oil
- 4 large red bell peppers, diced
- 4 teaspoons Hungarian paprika
- 1 teaspoon ground cardamom
- 4 cups vegetable broth or water
- 4 tablespoons whipping cream
- 1 large onion, diced
- 2-4 fresh green Thai or Serrano chili peppers, coarsely chopped
- Salt to taste
- 1 cup shelled pistachio nuts
- 2 cups nonfat buttermilk
- ½ cup finely chopped fresh cilantro or basil

Directions:

1. Place a soup pot over medium heat. Add oil. When the oil is heated, add onion, chili and bell pepper and sauté until onion is light brown.
2. Add cardamom, salt and paprika and sauté for a few seconds until aromatic.
3. Add pistachio and water. When it begins to boil, lower the heat and cover with a lid. Cook until the vegetables are tender. Turn off the heat.
4. Cool for a while and transfer into a blender. Blend until smooth. Pour the soup back into the pot.
5. Place the pot over medium heat.
6. Add buttermilk and cream into a bowl and whisk well. Add into the soup. Mix well. Do not boil. When the soup is well heated, turn off the heat.
7. Ladle into soup bowls and serve garnished with cilantro.

Turmeric Chicken Stew

Serves: 3

Ingredients:

- 1 tablespoon olive oil
- 1 sweet potato, cubed
- 1 medium eggplant, cubed
- ½ tablespoon minced fresh ginger
- ¼ cup low sodium chicken broth
- 1 chicken breast, skinless, boneless, cubed
- 1 small red onion, chopped
- 1 clove garlic, minced
- 1 teaspoon turmeric powder

Directions:

1. Place a skillet over medium-high heat. Add oil. When the oil is heated, add chicken and sear until browned.
2. Stir in the onion and sweet potato and cook until onion turns pink.
3. Stir in garlic, eggplant, ginger and turmeric and sauté for a few seconds until aromatic.
4. Add broth and simmer until the desired thickness is achieved. Stir occasionally.
5. Ladle into bowls and serve.

No-Chop Skillet Chili

Serves: 8

Ingredients:

- 2 teaspoons canola oil
- 2 cans (15 ounces each) unsalted red kidney beans, rinsed, drained
- 2 packages (14.4 ounces each) frozen sweet pepper and onion stir-fry vegetables
- 4-6 teaspoons chili powder
- 24 ounces 95% lean ground beef
- 2 cans (14 1/2 ounces each) unsalted diced tomatoes, with its liquid
- 2 packages (1 1/4 ounces each) low sodium taco seasoning or chili seasoning
- 4 tablespoons ketchup

To serve: Use any one or more
- Low fat shredded Cheddar cheese
- Black olives, sliced
- Plain fat free Greek yogurt
- Green onions, sliced
- Chopped cilantro

Directions:

1. Place a cast iron skillet over high heat. Add beef and sauté until brown. Break it simultaneously as it cooks.
2. Add rest of the ingredients except ketchup and stir.
3. Lower the heat and cover with a lid. Simmer until the vegetables are cooked.
4. Turn off the heat. Add ketchup and stir. Cover and let it sit for a while.
5. Ladle into bowls. Top with the suggested toppings and serve.

Chapter 9 - Lunch Recipes

Protein Packed Tuna Salad Pitas

Serves: 4

Ingredients:

- 4 whole wheat pitas
- Juice of a lemon
- 1 small onion, diced
- 2 tablespoons chopped parsley
- 2 cans tuna packed in water, unsalted
- 4 tablespoons olive oil
- 1 cup chopped red bell pepper
- Salt to taste
- Pepper to taste

Directions:

1. Add tuna, lemon juice, oil, bell pepper, parsley and onion into a bowl and toss. Add salt and pepper to taste.
2. Fill into the pitas and serve.

Green Pizza

Serves: 3

Ingredients:

- ½ pound prepared whole wheat pizza dough
- 2 tablespoons water
- Salt to taste
- ½ cup prepared pesto
- 1 cup chopped broccoli florets
- 2 1/2 ounces arugula, discard hard stems, chopped (about 3 cups)
- Freshly ground pepper to taste
- ½ cup part- skim Mozzarella cheese

Directions:

1. Place rack in the bottommost position in the oven.
2. Grease a baking sheet with cooking spray.
3. Dust your countertop with a little flour. Roll the dough, to the preferred thickness and place on the baking sheet.
4. Bake in a preheated oven at 450°F for 8-10 minutes.
5. Add broccoli and water into a saucepan. Place saucepan over medium heat. Cook until broccoli is crisp as well as tender. Add arugula and cook for a minute. Add salt and pepper to taste. Turn off the heat.
6. Smear the baked pizza crust with pesto. Scatter broccoli mixture on top.
7. Top with cheese.
8. Bake until crisp and the cheese melts.

White Bean Wrap

Serves: 2

Ingredients:

- 1 tablespoon apple cider vinegar
- 1 teaspoon finely chopped canned chipotle chili in adobo sauce
- 1 cup shredded red cabbage
- 2 tablespoons chopped fresh cilantro
- 1 small ripe avocado, peeled, pitted, chopped
- 1 tablespoon minced red onion
- ½ tablespoon canola oil
- Salt to taste
- 1 small carrot, shredded
- ½ can (from a 15 ounces can) white beans, rinsed
- ¼ cup shredded Sharp Cheddar cheese
- 2 whole wheat wraps or tortillas (8-10 inches each)

Directions:

1. Add vinegar, chipotle chili, oil and salt into a bowl and whisk well.
2. Add the vegetables and toss well.
3. Add beans and avocado into another bowl and mash until desired consistency.
4. Add cheese and onion and mix well.
5. Spread the wraps on your countertop. Spread about ½ cup of the bean mixture on the wraps. Scatter cabbage mixture. Roll like a burrito. Wrap in foil if desired and serve.

Cheesesteak Stuffed Peppers

Serves: 2

Ingredients:

- 2 bell peppers, halved
- 1 medium onion, sliced
- Kosher salt to taste
- ¾ pound sirloin steak, thinly sliced
- 8 slices provolone cheese
- ½ tablespoon vegetable oil
- 8 ounces cremini mushrooms, sliced
- Freshly ground black pepper to taste
- 1 teaspoon Italian seasoning or more to taste
- A handful fresh parsley, chopped

Directions:

1. Deseed the pepper halves and place in a baking dish.
2. Bake in a preheated oven at 325° F for about 20 minutes.
3. Place a skillet over medium heat. Add oil and heat. Add onions, salt, pepper and mushrooms and sauté until tender. Sprinkle salt and pepper over the steak and add into the skillet. Cook for 3 minutes. Stir a couple of times while cooking.
4. Add Italian seasoning and stir,
5. Place a provolone slice in each bell pepper half. Fill with steak mixture. Place another provolone slice on top of the steak mixture.
6. Set the oven to broiler mode. Broil until cheese melts and golden brown on top.
7. Sprinkle parsley on top and serve.

Couscous with Zucchini & Cherry Tomatoes

Serves: 8-10

Ingredients:

- 2 teaspoons olive oil
- 2 cloves garlic, minced
- 24 ounces zucchini
- ½ teaspoon salt
- 1 ½ cups whole wheat couscous
- 2 small onions, thinly sliced into rounds, separate the rings
- A handful of fresh thyme, chopped
- A few thyme sprigs, to garnish
- 2 cups halved cherry tomatoes

Directions:

1. Cut each zucchini into 3 pieces, crosswise. Next cut each piece into ½ inch thick wedges, lengthwise.
2. Place a large saucepan over medium heat. Add oil and let it heat. Add onion and garlic and sauté until golden brown.
3. Stir in the broth and bring to a boil.
4. Add zucchini, chopped thyme and salt and sauté until zucchini is crisp as well as tender.
5. Add tomatoes and couscous and stir. Turn off the heat. Cover and let it sit for a few minutes until dry.
6. Fluff the couscous with a fork. Cool for a few minutes.
7. Scatter thyme sprigs on top and serve.

Black Bean Quesadillas

Serves: 2

Ingredients:

- ½ can (from a 15 ounces can) black beans, rinsed, drained
- ¼ cup prepared salsa, divided
- 1 teaspoon canola oil, divided
- ¼ cup Monterey Jack cheese, preferably pepper Jack cheese
- 2 whole wheat tortillas (8 inches each)
- 1 small ripe avocado, peeled, pitted, chopped

Directions:

1. Add beans, 2 tablespoons salsa and cheese into a bowl and stir.
2. Spread the tortillas on your countertop. Divide the bean filling equally and spread it on one half of the tortillas. Fold the other half over the filling. Press gently to spread the filling.
3. Place a non-stick pan over medium heat. Add half the oil and swirl the pan to spread the oil. Place the quesadilla on the pan and cook until the underside is golden brown. Flip sides and cook the other side until golden brown.
4. Repeat the previous step and fry the other quesadilla.
5. Serve with avocado and a tablespoon of salsa.

Caprese Zoodles

Serves: 2

Ingredients:

- 2 large zucchinis
- Salt to taste
- 1 cup halved cherry tomatoes
- 2 tablespoons chopped fresh basil leaves
- 1 tablespoon extra-virgin olive oil
- ½ cup mozzarella balls, halved or quartered depending on the size
- 1 tablespoon balsamic vinegar

Directions:

1. Make noodles of the zucchini using a spiralizer or julienne peeler.
2. Add noodles into a bowl. Drizzle oil over it. Sprinkle salt and pepper and toss well.
3. Add rest of the ingredients and toss well.
4. Serve immediately.

Blackened Shrimp Bowls

Serves: 2

Ingredients:

- ½ pound shrimp, discard tails, peeled, deveined
- ½ teaspoon paprika
- 1 teaspoon onion powder
- Freshly ground pepper to taste
- ½ cup fire roasted corn
- 1 tablespoon chopped cilantro + extra to garnish
- 1 small avocado, peeled, pitted, sliced
- 1 cup cooked brown rice
- 1 teaspoon ground cumin
- ½ teaspoon garlic powder
- Kosher salt to taste
- 1 tablespoon olive oil, divided
- ½ red pepper, diced
- Juice of ½ lime, divided

Directions:

1. For shrimp: Add shrimp into a bowl. Sprinkle all the spices and salt over it. Toss well.
2. Place a skillet over medium-high heat. Add half the oil. When the oil is heated, add shrimp and cook until it turns translucent and charred as well.
3. For salad: Add corn, red pepper and cilantro into a bowl and toss.
4. Drizzle remaining oil, lime juice, salt and pepper over it and toss well.
5. To assemble: Add ½ cup rice into each bowl. Layer with shrimp followed by corn salad and finally avocado slices.
6. Sprinkle cilantro on top and drizzle lime juice and serve.

Black Bean & Salmon Tostadas

Serves: 2 (2 tostadas per serving)

Ingredients:

- 4 corn tortillas (6 inches each)
- ½ can (from a 6-7 ounces can) skinless wild Alaskan salmon, drained
- 1 tablespoon minced pickled jalapeños
- 1 tablespoon pickling juice
- 1 tablespoon chopped cilantro
- 1 ½ tablespoons low fat sour cream
- 1 scallion, chopped
- ½ avocado, peeled, pitted, chopped
- 1 ½ tablespoons reduced fat sour cream
- 1 scallion, chopped
- 1 tablespoon prepared salsa
- ½ can (from a 15 ounces can)
- Lime wedges to serve (optional)
- Cooking spray

Directions:

1. Place tortillas on a large baking sheet. Spray some cooking spray over it.
2. Bake in a preheated oven at 450°F for 12-14 minutes or until light brown.
3. Add salmon, avocado and jalapeño into a bowl and toss well.
4. Add black beans, salsa, sour cream and scallions into the food processor bowl and process until smooth.
5. Spoon into a microwave safe bowl. Microwave on high for 1-2 minutes until well heated.
6. To assemble: Place the tortillas on individual serving plates. Spread the bean mixture on each tortilla.
7. Top with salmon mixture and cabbage salad and serve with lime wedges.

Taco Tomatoes

Serves: 8

Ingredients:

- 2 tablespoons extra virgin olive oil
- 2 medium onions, chopped
- 8 large ripe beefsteak tomatoes
- 1 cup shredded iceberg lettuce
- 1 ½ pounds ground beef
- 2 packets (1 ounce each) taco seasoning
- 1 cup shredded Mexican cheese blend
- ½ cup sour cream

Directions:

1. Place a large skillet over medium heat. Add oil and let it heat. Add onion and sauté until translucent.
2. Stir in the beef and taco seasoning. Cook until meat is not pink anymore. Break it simultaneously as it cooks. Turn off the heat. Discard the fat remaining in the pan.
3. Place the tomatoes on your cutting board, with the stem side facing down.
4. Cut 6 wedges of each tomato. Go up to ¾ the tomato. Do not separate the wedges. The tomato should be intact at the stem area.
5. Carefully open the wedges (like the petals of a flower). Divide the meat equally and place in the tomatoes. Sprinkle cheese and lettuce over the meat.
6. Drizzle sour cream and serve.

Lemon-Garlic Chicken Drumsticks

Serves: 2-3

Ingredients:

- 5-6 skin-on chicken drumsticks
- 2 tablespoons butter
- Zest of ½ lemon
- Juice of ½ lemon
- Salt to taste
- Freshly ground pepper to taste
- ½ tablespoon olive oil
- 2 cloves garlic, finely chopped
- 1 tablespoon parsley, chopped, to garnish

Directions:

1. Sprinkle salt and pepper over the chicken drumsticks. Place in a bowl. Set aside for 30-40 minutes.
2. Place a heavy bottomed skillet over medium-high heat. Add oil and 1 tablespoon butter and let it melt.
3. Add chicken drumsticks and cook until browned all over.
4. Lower the heat to medium-low. Cover with a lid and cook for about 20 minutes. Turn the chicken every few minutes.
5. Add rest of the ingredients and toss well. Turn off the heat. Cover and let it sit for 5 minutes.
6. Garnish with parsley and serve.

Cheddar-Stuffed Mini Meatloaves with Chipotle Glaze

Serves: 2

Ingredients:

- ½ pound 90% lean ground beef
- 3 tablespoons fine, dry whole-wheat breadcrumbs
- 3 tablespoons ketchup
- ½ teaspoon ground cumin
- Freshly ground pepper to taste
- 1/8 teaspoon ground chipotle pepper
- 1 small onion, finely chopped
- 1 small egg
- 1 teaspoon chili powder
- Salt to taste
- ¼ cup shredded extra-sharp Cheddar cheese
- Cooking spray

Directions:

1. Grease 2 small baking dishes or mini loaf pans with cooking spray. Place them on a baking sheet.
2. Set aside cheese, chipotle chili and 2 tablespoons of ketchup and add rest of the ingredients into a bowl. Mix well.
3. Divide equally and place in the prepared pans. Using your finger, make a deep cut of about 1-½ inches along the central line on top of the meatloaves. Sprinkle cheese a tablespoon of cheese in this indentation in each of the meatloaves. . Press the edges of the cuts together so that the cheese remains stuffed in the meatloaves.
4. Add chipotle chili and 2 tablespoons ketchup into a bowl and stir. Brush this mixture on top of the meatloaves.
5. Place the meatloaves along with the baking sheet in a preheated oven.

6. Bake at 450° F for 20-30 minutes or until a meat thermometer when inserted in the centre of the meatloaves shows 165° F.
7. Serve warm.

Chapter 10 - Dinner Recipes

Peanut Chicken with Veggies and Rice
Serves: 2
Ingredients:
<u>For peanut sauce:</u>
- 3 tablespoons creamy peanut butter
- ½ tablespoon fresh lime juice
- ½ tablespoon minced ginger
- 1 teaspoon honey
- ¼ teaspoon red pepper flakes or more to taste + extra to garnish
- ½ tablespoon sesame oil
- 1 clove garlic, minced
- ½ tablespoon low-sodium soy sauce
- 2-3 tablespoons water

<u>For chicken and stir fry vegetables:</u>
- 1 cup cooked, shredded chicken
- 1 ½ cups chopped broccoli florets
- 1 medium carrot, peeled, cut into 1/8 inch thick rounds
- ½ cup shelled edamame, fresh or frozen
- ½ tablespoon minced ginger
- ½ tablespoon extra-virgin olive oil
- 1 large red bell pepper, thinly sliced
- 2-3 green onions, sliced, separate the white and green parts
- 1 clove garlic, minced
- ½ tablespoon low sodium soy sauce

<u>To serve:</u>
- Cooked brown rice or quinoa or brown rice noodles or soba noodles
- 1 green onion, thinly sliced
- Toasted sesame seeds

- Red pepper flakes

Directions:
1. To make peanut sauce: Add all the ingredients for peanut sauce into a saucepan.
2. Place saucepan over medium heat. Add some more water if you would like to dilute the sauce.
3. Add chicken and stir. Remove from heat. Cover and set aside.
4. To make stir fry vegetables: Place a nonstick skillet over medium high heat. Add oil and heat.
5. Add bell pepper, broccoli, carrots, white and light green parts of the green onion and sauté until crisp as well as tender.
6. Stir in rest of the ingredients for stir fry vegetables. Toss until well coated.
7. Stir fry until the vegetables are crisp as well as tender.
8. Stir in edamame, garlic, soy sauce, ginger and onion greens and toss until well coated. Turn off the heat.
9. To assemble: Add rice into serving bowls. Layer with vegetables followed by peanut chicken and the suggested toppings and serve.

Harvest Chicken Casserole

Serves: 3-4

Ingredients:

- 1 tablespoon extra-virgin olive oil + extra to grease
- Kosher salt to taste
- 1 small onion, chopped
- ½ pound Brussels sprouts, trimmed, quartered
- 1 pound skinless, boneless chicken breasts
- Freshly ground pepper to taste
- 1 medium sweet potato, peeled, cut into small cubes
- ½ teaspoon dried thyme
- 2 tablespoons chicken broth
- ¼ cup dried cranberries
- 1 medium sweet potato, peeled, cut into small cubes
- ½ teaspoon dried thyme
- 3 cups cooked wild rice
- ¼ cup sliced almonds

Directions:

1. Place a deep skillet over medium-high heat. Add half the oil and let it heat.
2. Sprinkle salt and pepper over the chicken and place in the skillet.
3. Cook until golden. Flip sides and cook the other side until golden brown.
4. Remove with a slotted spoon and place on your cutting board. When cool enough to handle, chop into bite size pieces.
5. Add remaining oil into the skillet. When the oil is heated, add sweet potato, onion and Brussels sprouts and stir.
6. Stir in thyme, salt, paprika and pepper and cook until soft.

7. Stir in the broth and cover with a lid. Cook until sweet potato is soft.
8. Add rice, cranberries and chicken and mix well. Transfer into a greased baking dish. Sprinkle almonds on top.
9. Bake in a preheated oven at 325° F for about 20 minutes.
10. Remove from the oven and cool for 5 minutes.
11. Serve.

Stir-Fried Pork with Ginger and Soy Sauce

Serves: 4

Ingredients:

- 18 ounces pork tenderloin, trimmed of fat, chopped into bite size pieces
- 4 tablespoons dark soy sauce
- 11 ounces button mushrooms, sliced
- 5 ounces mangetout, trimmed
- 2 cloves garlic, peeled, thinly sliced
- Freshly ground pepper to taste
- 2 teaspoons corn-starch
- ¼ cup water
- 4 red bell peppers, deseeded, sliced
- 2 inches ginger, peeled, cut into thin matchsticks
- 8 spring onions, cut into 1 inch pieces
- Cooking spray

Directions:

1. Place a large wok over high heat. Spray with cooking spray. Sprinkle salt and pepper over pork and add into the heated wok.
2. Cook until browned all over. Remove onto a plate.
3. Spray the wok with some more oil. Add mushrooms and peppers and sauté for a couple of minutes.
4. Stir in mangetout and sauté for a minute.
5. Stir in garlic, ginger and spring onions and cook until aromatic.
6. Add pork back into the pot.
7. Whisk together cornstarch, soy sauce and water in a bowl and pour into the wok.
8. Stir constantly until mixture thickens. Cook until the pork is cooked to the desired doneness.
9. Serve right away.

Broccoli, Beef & Potato Hot dish

Serves: 4

Ingredients:

- ¾ pound broccoli, cut into 1 inch florets
- ¾ pound 95% lean ground beef
- 1 tablespoon Worcestershire sauce
- Salt to taste
- 3 tablespoons corn-starch
- 1/8 teaspoon turmeric powder
- 1 small egg, lightly beaten
- 1/8 teaspoon Hungarian paprika
- 1 tablespoon canola oil, divided
- 1 medium onion, chopped
- ½ teaspoon garlic powder
- 2 cups low-fat milk
- Freshly ground pepper to taste
- 1 cup shredded Sharp Cheddar cheese, preferably orange
- 2 cups frozen hash-brown or precooked shredded potatoes
- Canola or olive oil cooking spray

Directions:

1. Place broccoli in a bowl. Drizzle ½ tablespoon oil over it. Toss well and transfer onto a baking sheet. Spread it in a single layer.
2. Roast in a preheated oven at 450° F for about 15-20 minutes or brown at a few places.
3. Add remaining oil into the skillet. When the oil is heated, add beef and onion and cook until brown. Break it simultaneously as it cooks.
4. Add Worcestershire sauce, salt and garlic powder and mix well. Turn off the heat and transfer into a baking dish.

5. Add milk and cornstarch into a saucepan and whisk well. Place saucepan over medium-high heat.
6. Stir constantly until thick. When it coats the back of a spoon, turn off the heat. Add Cheddar cheese, turmeric and salt and mix well. Stir constantly until cheese melts.
7. Pour cheese sauce over the beef mixture. Scatter broccoli on top.
8. Add egg, hash-browns, salt and pepper into a bowl and mix well. Spread it over the broccoli. Spray with cooking spray.
9. Bake in a preheated oven at 400° F for about 20-30 minutes or brown at a few places.
10. Remove from the oven and garnish with paprika. Cool for 10 minutes and serve.

Creamy Garlic Pasta with Shrimp & Vegetables

Serves: 2

Ingredients:

- 3 ounces whole-wheat spaghetti
- ½ bunch asparagus, trimmed, thinly sliced
- ½ cup fresh or frozen peas
- Salt to taste
- 2 tablespoons chopped flat-leaf parsley
- ½ tablespoon extra-virgin olive oil
- 2 tablespoons toasted pine nuts
- 6 ounces peeled, deveined, raw shrimp, cut into 1 inch pieces
- 1 medium red bell pepper, thinly sliced
- 2 cloves garlic, chopped
- ¾ cup non-fat or low-fat plain yogurt
- 1 ½ tablespoons lemon juice
- Freshly ground pepper to taste

Directions:

1. Cook the spaghetti following the directions on the package but for 2 minutes less than the specified time.
2. Add asparagus, shrimp, peas and bell pepper and cook until pasta is al dente. Drain and set aside.
3. Add garlic and salt into a bowl and mash with the back of a spoon until a paste is formed.
4. Add yogurt lemon juice, pepper, parsley and oil into a bowl and whisk well.
5. Add pasta mixture and fold gently.
6. Garnish with pine nuts and serve.

Pan-Fried Tilapia

Serves: 2

Ingredients:

- ½ cup corn-starch or almond flour
- ½ teaspoon onion powder
- ½ teaspoon garlic powder
- ¼ teaspoon ground cumin
- ½ teaspoon chili powder
- 2 tilapia fillets (6 ounces each)
- Freshly ground pepper to taste
- Salt to taste
- 1 tablespoon fresh cilantro leaves, to garnish
- ½ tablespoon canola oil or vegetable oil
- Lime wedges to serve

Directions:

1. Add all the dry ingredients into a bowl and stir.
2. Sprinkle salt and pepper over the fillets. Dredge the fillets in the dry ingredients mixture. Shake to drop off extra mixture and place on a plate.
3. Place a nonstick skillet over medium heat. Add oil. When the oil is heated, add fillets and cook until the underside is golden brown. Flip sides and cook the other side until golden brown.
4. Serve garnished with cilantro and with lime wedges.

Chermoula Tofu and Roasted Vegetables

Serves: 2

Ingredients:

For chermoula tofu:

- 2 tablespoons finely chopped cilantro
- ½ teaspoon cumin seeds, lightly crushed
- ¼ teaspoon crushed dried chilies or more to taste
- 4 1/2 ounces tofu
- 2 cloves garlic, chopped
- Zest of ½ lemon, grated
- ½ tablespoon olive oil

For roasted vegetables:

- 1 red onion, quartered
- 1 yellow bell pepper, deseeded, sliced
- 1 red bell pepper, deseeded, sliced
- 1 courgette, thickly sliced
- 2 small eggplants, thickly sliced
- Salt to taste
- Cooking spray

Directions:

1. Add all the ingredients for chermoula except tofu into a bowl and stir.
2. Dry the tofu by patting with paper towels.
3. Cut the tofu into thin slices and place on a plate. Divide the chermoula among the slices and spread it evenly over it.
4. Spread the vegetables in a baking dish. Spray with cooking spray.
5. Roast in a preheated oven at 400° F for about 20-30 minutes or brown at a few places. Stir the vegetables a couple of times while cooking.
6. Place tofu slices over the vegetables, with the chermoula side facing up.
7. Bake for 15 minutes.

8. Divide into 2 plates and serve.

Broccoli Rabe, White Bean & Fontina Pasta

Serves: 2

Ingredients:

- 4 ounces whole-wheat pasta shells, fusilli or chiocciole
- ¾ cup vegetable broth or chicken broth
- 1 tablespoon extra-virgin olive oil
- ½ can (from a 19 ounces can) cannellini beans, rinsed
- Salt to taste
- ¼ cup toasted breadcrumbs
- 1 medium bunch broccoli rabe, trimmed, cut into 1 inch pieces or 4 cups baby spinach
- ½ tablespoon all-purpose flour
- 2 cloves garlic, minced
- 1 tablespoon red wine vinegar
- Freshly ground pepper to taste
- 1/3 cup shredded Fontina cheese

Directions:

1. Cook pasta following the directions on the package. Add broccoli rabe during the last 2 minutes of cooking. Drain and set aside.
2. Add broth and flour in a small bowl and whisk well.
3. Place a skillet over medium heat. Add oil. When the oil is heated, add garlic and sauté until aromatic. Add the flour mixture and stir constantly until thick.
4. Stir in beans, vinegar, beans and seasoning.
5. Add pasta and broccoli rabe and heat thoroughly. Turn off the heat.
6. Add cheese and stir until cheese is melted.
7. Garnish with toasted breadcrumbs and serve.

Vegetarian Shepherd's Pies

Serves: 2

Ingredients:

- ½ pound Yukon gold or white potatoes, peeled, cubed
- ½ tablespoon butter
- Freshly ground pepper to taste
- 1 medium onion, finely chopped
- 1/3 -½ cup frozen corn kernels, thawed
- 1 ½ tablespoons all-purpose flour
- ¾ cup cooked or canned lentils
- ¼ cup buttermilk
- Salt to taste
- ½ tablespoon extra-virgin olive oil
- ¼ cup finely diced carrots
- ¼ teaspoon dried thyme
- 2 teaspoons water
- 7 ounces vegetable broth
- Cooking spray

Directions:

1. Add potatoes into a saucepan. Pour enough water to cover the potatoes.
2. Place saucepan over medium heat. Cover with a lid partially and cook until soft.
3. Drain and add the potatoes back into the saucepan. Add butter, buttermilk, salt and pepper and mash until smooth using a potato masher.
4. Meanwhile, place rack in the upper third of the oven. Set the oven to broiler mode.
5. Grease 2 ramekins with cooking spray. Place the ramekins on a baking sheet.
6. Place a skillet over medium-high heat. Add oil. When the oil is heated, add onion and carrot and stir. Add water and cover with a lid.
7. Cook until slightly soft.

8. Add corn, salt, pepper and thyme and stir. Cook for a couple of minutes.
9. Dust with flour and mix well. Add broth and stir constantly until thick.
10. Add lentils and bring to a simmer. Cook for 2-3 minutes until nearly dry.
11. Add lentil mixture into the ramekins. Place mashed potatoes on top.
12. Place in a preheated oven and broil until light brown on top. Rotate the ramekins a couple of times while broiling.

Zucchini Manicotti

Serves: 2

Ingredients:

- ¾ cup Ricotta cheese
- 1 small egg, lightly beaten
- ¼ teaspoon Italian seasoning
- Freshly ground pepper to taste
- ½ cup marinara sauce
- 1 tablespoon thinly sliced fresh basil
- ½ cup finely grated Parmesan cheese, divided
- 2 cloves garlic, peeled, minced
- Kosher salt to taste
- 2 zucchini, cut into ¼ inch thick slices
- ¾ cup shredded Mozzarella cheese

Directions:

1. Grease a baking dish with cooking spray.
2. Add Ricotta, egg, Italian seasoning, ¼ cup Parmesan cheese, salt, pepper and garlic into a bowl and mix well.
3. Place 3 slices of zucchini, slightly overlapping each other. Place a heaping teaspoonful of the Ricotta mixture on the topmost zucchini slice. Roll the zucchini, starting from the filling side and place in the baking dish with the seam side facing down.
4. Spread marinara sauce over the zucchini manicotti. Top with remaining Parmesan cheese and Mozzarella cheese.
5. Bake in a preheated oven at 350° F for about 20-30 minutes or cheese melts and brown at a few places.
6. Cool for 5 minutes and serve garnished with basil

Conclusion

Thanks for buying this book. I hope that through the information presented here, you have learned much about the 5:2 intermittent fasting protocol to take the next important steps. After all, knowledge is just half the battle for a fitter and healthier you. The other half is application of knowledge or acting upon knowledge gained. So, act as soon as possible if you want to experience the health and weight-loss benefits of the 5:2 intermittent fasting protocol.

Here's to your health and fitness my friend. Cheers!

Let Us Help You Discover the Perfect Fasting Protocol for You

Much has been said about Intermittent Fasting. Yet, the bigger fraction of today's population has been unable to fully experience the power of this ancient natural health and wellness technique.

Many are unable to participate in this life changing experience because they do not know how to make it work for them.

Generally, getting the best out of Intermittent Fasting depends largely on understanding the best fasting protocol for you.

We are going to help you find the most suitable fasting protocol for you to begin your journey. All you need to do is email us your current eating schedule. Also let us know if you currently follow a fasting protocol or have experience with Intermittent Fasting. We will give you our feedback and suggestions for where you need to begin.

Email: smartnourishmentfast@gmail.com

References:

1. https://www.livestrong.com/article/438695-how-eat-stop-eat-works/
2. https://idmprogram.com/fed-fasted-state/
3. https://greatist.com/eat/intermittent-fasting-health-benefits-and-side-effects
4. https://www.dietspotlight.com/eat-stop-eat-review/
5. https://www.healthline.com/nutrition/10-health-benefits-of-intermittent-fasting#section9
6. https://www.healthline.com/health/how-to-exercise-safely-intermittent-fasting#6
7. https://defendyourhealthcare.us/exercises-for-the-eat-stop-eat-diet
8. https://personalexcellence.co/blog/fasting-success/

Made in the USA
Columbia, SC
13 April 2020